# URBAN PLANNING AND
# PUBLIC HEALTH IN AFRICA

T0299797

*To the memory of my brothers:*
*Fon Palma Njoh; Mukwa Nathanael Njoh; Ndah George Njoh;*
*Tah Ebenezer Njoh; and Nih Divine Njoh, who passed on in that order.*

# Urban Planning and Public Health in Africa
## Historical, Theoretical and Practical Dimensions of a Continent's Water and Sanitation Problematic

AMBE J. NJOH
*University of South Florida, USA*

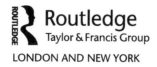

Routledge
Taylor & Francis Group

LONDON AND NEW YORK

First published 2012 by Ashgate Publishing

Published 2016 by Routledge
2 Park Square, Milton Park, Abingdon, Oxon OX14 4RN
711 Third Avenue, New York, NY 10017, USA

First issued in paperback 2017

*Routledge is an imprint of the Taylor & Francis Group, an informa business*

**British Library Cataloguing in Publication Data**
Njoh, Ambe J.
  Urban planning and public health in Africa : historical, theoretical and practical dimensions of a continent's water and sanitation problematic.
  1. City planning--Health aspects--Africa. 2. Urban health--Africa.
  3. Urban sanitation--Africa.
  I. Title
  363.7'2'096'091732-dc23

**Library of Congress Cataloging-in-Publication Data**
Njoh, Ambe J.
 Urban planning and public health in Africa : historical, theorectical and practical dimensions of a continent's water and sanitation problematic / by Ambe J. Njoh.
    p. cm.
  Includes bibliographical references and index.
  ISBN 978-1-4094-4318-6 (hbk)
 1. Urban health--Africa. 2. City planning--Health aspects--Africa.
 3. Public health--Africa. I. Title.
  RA566.5.A35N55 2012
  362.1096--dc23

                                                                    2012006634

ISBN 13: 978-1-138-10920-9 (pbk)
ISBN 13: 978-1-4094-4318-6 (hbk)

# Contents

# List of Figures, Tables and Boxes

## Figures

## Tables

**Boxes**

# Acknowledgements

Large-scale projects such as books can hardly be the product of anyone working solo. This particular piece of work is no exception. The idea of taking on the project is rooted in my contribution to the United Nations (UN) project under the caption, *Global Report on Human Settlement 2009: Planning Sustainable Cities*. As I completed the chapter on "The Emergence and Spread of Contemporary Urban Planning," the question of 'context' emerged as one that is important but oft-ignored in planning. In the process, the fact that urban planning and public health are professional cousins that have drifted apart, also caught my attention. The two professions emerged to address the negative externalities of the Industrial Revolution. My contribution to that project, as it is customary for work of that genre, was subjected to serious peer scrutiny. The contribution, and therefore the present book benefited immensely from the input of the brilliant colleagues with whom I collaborated on the project. I hasten to register my sincere thanks to said colleagues even though they may be unaware of their, albeit, indirect contribution to making this book a reality. I acknowledge my debt of gratitude to the editor of *Cities: The International Journal of Urban Policy and Planning*. His comments and those of three anonymous peer-reviewers of the article version of Chapter 9 were invaluable in my efforts to refine that chapter. I am also indebted to my colleagues at the University of South Florida. Particularly, I would like to thank the colleagues and students who attended my talks on public health implications of urban planning. The talks took place respectively at the Environmental Research and Interdisciplinary Colloquium, College of Public Health, and the Department of Geography, Environment and Planning Colloquium in Fall 2010. Their thoughtful and insightful questions helped me to refine some of the ideas I have expressed in this book.

I am indebted to all members of the Njoh family in Cameroon and the diaspora. The following deserve special mention: my wife, Fri, and children, Eni, Fon, Akwi, Nji, and Tenguh; my brother, Adig, and wife, Fuzie and children, Alex, Mah, Afor, Abang, Anne, and Azie; my sister, Akwi and niece, Yemi; my brother Muki, and son, Azobo. Many thanks to my uncle, Ni Fomunyoh Peter Azobo and family.

While I thank everyone who helped in the process of realizing this book, I take full responsibility for all errors contained therein.

# Preface

Established indicators of development suggest that, as a group, African countries lag behind their counterparts in other regions with respect to public health. Particularly noteworthy is the fact that the public health problems of these countries are rooted in preventable causes associated with hygiene and sanitation. Poor hygiene and sanitation conditions continue to constitute a leading cause of ill-health, poverty and commensurate problems in African countries.

This book highlights the nature of these problems. Evidence presented in the book suggests that, as a continent, Africa has the lowest sanitation coverage in the world. The lack or scarcity of clean water causes water-borne illnesses. Limited or no access to safe hygiene and sanitation facilities constitutes the primary cause of diarrhea, dysentery, and typhoid among others. In fact, the dearth or absence of such facilities has been identified as a leading cause of death among children under five. Malaria, a disease born of the anopheles mosquito, remains lethal, and a leading cause of death on the continent.

It is customary to attribute the problems that ail Africa to the lack of financial resources. This book deviates from convention by suggesting non-financial factors as the source of sanitation problems on the continent. For instance, combating malaria may require simply eliminating mosquito breeding grounds in the built environment. In practice this may entail no more than ridding human settlements of shrubbery and standing water. People can be sensitized to carry out these activities on their own without any financial input from the government. The linkages among factors at the root of many sanitation-related ailments in Africa are well known. For example, the incrimination of the anopheles mosquito as the vector of the parasite that causes malaria occurred more than a century ago. This book contends that the sanitation problems of African countries result mainly from institutional factors. Authorities in these countries are wedded to modernist urban planning models, which advocate conventional technology. The book sees such technology as unsustainable. It underscores a need to ensure that hygiene and sanitation technology is sustainable from socio-cultural and economic perspectives.

Yet, three questions remain unclear, and constitute prominent contributors to public health problems on the continent today. The first has to do with the role of urban planning as a tool of public health. In fact, there are questions about who has responsibility over public health. Is public health the exclusive domain of public health officials? Do other professionals such as urban planners, under whose auspices order in built space falls, have a role to play in promoting public health? This book answers these questions in the affirmative. It sees a critical role for urban planners in implementing public health policies within any given polity. Certainly extant building codes, the urban planner's domain, throughout Africa already contain public health elements. However, as a colonial legacy, the codes are anachronistic and sought to address public health needs of the past.

The second perennial issue revolves around knowledge of the nature and magnitude of Africa's hygiene and sanitation problem. This problem has always been misrepresented. This was particularly true during the colonial era. At the time, there was a tendency to paint a false image of Africans as people without a sense of, or desire for, cleanliness. Also, there was a proclivity for considering Africans as immune to deadly diseases such as malaria. Such deliberate mischaracterization of the African health problematic gave colonial governments badly needed cover for public health policies, which targeted exclusively European enclaves. The third question has to do with the issue of sustainability. This issue appears to be most critical with respect to the strategies and technologies that must be summoned to deal with hygiene and sanitation problems. What institutional model (e.g., private versus public) should be adopted for the purpose of collecting and managing a city's wastes? What technologies should be adopted for the purpose of collecting, transporting and treating excreta and wastewater in any given setting?

Their importance notwithstanding, these questions have never been dealt with in a systematic, comprehensive and interrelated fashion. Thus, it would appear that their inextricably interconnected nature has largely eluded the attention of analysts. This book recognizes the crucial link among the various factors highlighted here and seeks to draw attention to the common thread linking them. A substantial part of the book looks into the past, especially because we are unlikely to know where we are going if we know not whence we come. It also spends much time painting a vivid picture of the hygiene and sanitation conditions characterizing different sub-regions of Africa. The importance of having some appreciation for these conditions cannot be overemphasized. If nothing else, highlighting the problems in their regional contexts serves to guard against the costly tendency of over-generalizing Africa's socio-economic problematic.

# Chapter 1
# A Brief History of Public Health and the Built Environment

**Introduction**

The importance of appreciating history cannot be overstated. History holds many lessons for today and the future. To be sure, our forebears encountered and attempted to resolve some of the same kind of problems we are faced with today. Therefore, it makes much sense in terms of the time, financial and other resources that can be potentially saved to simply borrow lessons of experience from our predecessors. There is no denying, as an old adage suggests, that those incapable of learning from history are doomed to repeat past mistakes. A synonymous adage avows that knowledge of one's origin is essential to accurately guess one's destination. The history of public health as a crucial element of human settlement development is very rich. Consequently, it holds many potentially useful lessons for contemporary town planning. One objective of this chapter is to summarize this history. The chapter has a secondary purpose, namely to introduce subsequent chapters and lay out a plan for the rest of the book.

**Urban planning and public health**

Several factors account for the failure to register more positive results in public health in Africa. Prominent among these is the tendency to stress the curative or treatment approach to dealing with health problems. One consequence of this is that preventative health measures tend to be ignored. This has not always been the case. From time immemorial public health, as its name suggests, has always recognized the need to prevent health-threatening conditions. The success of efforts to address this need was guaranteed by involving not only public health experts but also experts from other fields. In particular, as was the case in efforts to deal with the negative externalities of the industrial revolution, urban planning expertise was required. For a long time subsequent to the immediate post-industrial revolution era, public health officials and urban planners collaborated to protect public health. Since then, the two professions have drifted apart. Yet, the need for collaboration between the two professions has grown more compelling rather than diminishing.

This book underscores the role that urban planning can play in mitigating health-threatening conditions in Africa. Expertise in urban planning, more than in any other field, is necessary to prevent health threats and deaths resulting from the following.

- Malaria;
- Insalubrious conditions;
- Injuries in the built environment;
- Traffic accidents;
- Poverty.

*Malaria*

This is the leading cause of death in Africa. The anopheles mosquito has been incriminated as the vector of this deadly disease. A bite from an anopheles mosquito infected with the plasmodium parasite causes malaria in people and some animals. Africans, particularly those close to the equator, are at risk from the deadliest form of the plasmodium parasite, namely plasmodium falciparum *(P. falciparum)*. Although there are a few anti-malaria drugs, such as chloroquine, an effective vaccine against this disease is yet to be invented. Even when anti-malarial drugs are available, they are prohibitively expensive. Thus, the only sustainable means of preventing malaria to date are those targeting the mosquitoes constituting vectors of malaria. Although mosquito nets and insecticides find utility here, the most effective strategies in terms of cost and coverage involve urban planning and design. As discussed later, colonial authorities were patently aware of these strategies. Accordingly, they mandated the draining of standing water in human settlements as a mosquito-control measure. The highly controversial programme of locating exclusive European enclaves on high altitudes away from swampy areas was also intended to insulate Europeans from mosquitoes. Another measure that colonial authorities instituted to insulate people from mosquitoes in exclusive European enclaves was the fitting of all openings on housing units with screens. If these measures were controversial it is not because they were devoid of logic. Rather, they are controversial on ethical grounds. The measures were designed to protect exclusively the health of Europeans while ignoring that of Africans. Contemporary efforts to fend off malarial infections are guaranteed to be more effective if they institute measures to: 1) locate human settlements away from swamps; 2) drain all standing water in these settlements; and 3) fit all openings on housing units with screens.

*Insalubrious conditions*

An insalubrious environment is characterized by the indiscriminate disposal of waste. This waste may be of the domestic, human or industrial variety. Insalubrious conditions are at the root of lethal diseases such as dysentery, diarrhea, cholera, and tuberculosis. These diseases are among the leading causes of death in Africa. Contrary to conventional practices, curative or treatment-oriented strategies are less effective in dealing with these diseases than measures of the preventative variety. Urban planners are capable of helping to accomplish objectives requiring the latter. In this regard, planners can be summoned to develop robust but attainable and sustainable hygiene and sanitation standards governing residential and human settlement development. Such standards would invariably deal with issues including but not limited to, human waste disposal, the collection, handling and disposal of other types of waste, and systems for transporting, storing and distributing potable water.

*Injuries in the built environment*

Injuries in the built environment may be incurred indoors or outdoors. Indoor injuries may result from badly designed interior spaces. Poorly designed interior spaces may take the form of rooms, doors, and stairs with runs that are too narrow, for human use. Such designs may also assume the form of stairways that are too steep or very sharp internal turns, and inadequately lighted or unlit indoor spaces. When poorly designed, outdoor spaces can also contribute significantly to injuries in the built environment. Poorly designed outdoor space may take the form of buildings that are juxtaposed in a manner that fails to promote functionality. Such space may also manifest itself in failure to include facilities that permit the use of outdoor space by the physically or visually challenged. Sound legislation articulated in the form of building codes and spatial development standards would go a good way in eliminating such spaces.

*Traffic accidents*

Traffic accidents rank tenth among Africa's public health threats (Cooke, 2009). It is true that a substantial proportion of the accidents result from the incompetence of drivers and poorly maintained vehicles. However, most of the accidents result from poorly designed and poorly maintained roads. Victims of traffic accidents in built-up areas are often pedestrians who are compelled to share the carriageway with vehicular traffic because of the absence of sidewalks. This problem is compounded by the lack of street lights, inadequate or no street signage and no designated pedestrian crossings. Resolving these problems does not require expertise in public health. Rather, it requires expertise in urban planning.

*Poverty*

It is true that poverty, in and of itself, is not a disease. However, it is a public health issue to the extent that it is capable of affecting a person's well-being. Not only is poverty stressful, it prevents the afflicted from having access to the basic amenities of life such as livable housing, nutritious food, and potable water. This suggests that in efforts to deal with the health problems identified above, urban planners must be conscious of the need to alleviate poverty. Thus, for instance, alternative strategies for waste collection must be evaluated on the basis of their ability to contribute to poverty alleviation efforts. Similarly, decisions to improve sanitary conditions in inner cities cannot afford to be oblivious to the needs of the poor. In the past, authorities have, for instance, destroyed without replacing, housing units of poor people in the name of slum clearance. Urban planners are in a unique position, thanks to their expertise, to dissuade authorities from taking such ill-advised decisions. Before ending this subsection, it is necessary to underscore the following point.

This book focuses mainly on sanitation conditions and efforts to ameliorate these conditions in Africa in historical and contemporary perspectives. Yet, it is worth noting that health-threatening factors requiring urban planning interventions in the built environment are inextricably intertwined. Therefore, any discussion of one of these factors invariably invites more than passing mention of one or more cognate factors.

## Public health promotion in ancient human settlements

Many hygiene and sanitation problems of the past are reoccurring today. More noteworthy, as suggested earlier, is the fact that our predecessors found ways to address these problems. However, evidence of the strategies they employed in this regard is scant. George Rosen is among the few who have paid more than passing interest to questions of sanitation and hygiene in the ancient world. The first chapter of his book on the History of Public Health (1958) contains vivid accounts of health problems in ancient human settlements such as Kahun in Egypt, the Indus Valley in India, Mohenjo-Daro in the Indus Valley and Harapa in the Punjab. The accounts suggest that hygiene and sanitation problems have remained largely the same since ancient times. The same can, however, not be said of the strategies summoned to address the problems. While there are a few similarities here and there, contemporary strategies deviate significantly from ancient variants.

Let's begin by examining the similarities. Archaeological finds in ancient cities of India have revealed the presence of carefully planned cities complete with bathrooms, drainage and sewerage systems. There is also evidence attesting to efforts to regulate neighbourhood layout the physical arrangement of buildings. Part of these efforts were directed at controlling how and where wastes could be disposed of. Remarkably, and similar to the situation in contemporary cities, the drains were laid below the street surface at a depth of about 2 feet (60cm). In addition, the drains consisted of molded bricks bound together by clay mortar. Furthermore, the drain pipes were produced from pottery and laid in gypsum plaster to prevent leakage. Paradoxically, indoor plumbing, including such facilities as bathrooms, constituted part of the hygiene and sanitation systems of some ancient human settlements. The abodes of royal families and other notables such as the Knossos on Crete (circa, 2nd Christian Millennium) are said to have been furnished with toilet facilities, including bathrooms and flushable toilets

(Rosen, 1958). Further evidence in this regard was unveiled in Kahun and Tel-el-Amarna. Both cities existed around the fourteenth century B.C. Archaeological excavations in Priene in present-day Turkey, have uncovered evidence showing that water was drawn from public wells and distributed to private homes through pipes. Similar excavations in the same general area reveal that the ancient city of Troy was equipped with a sophisticated water supply system. Along the same lines, studies of ancient Cretan-Mycenean culture have unmasked remnants of what appear to be well-developed underground water conduits. Evidence of elaborate indoor sanitation services and meticulous sewerage systems have also been found in the ruins of Inca human settlements. Here too, the problem of water supply in human communities appeared to have essentially been solved.

From the foregoing narrative it is clear that sanitation and hygiene practices in the built environment are not new. Rather, such practices date back to antiquity. The historical connection between these phenomena is asserted more succinctly in the following words by Rosen (1958: 1):

> Throughout human history, the major problems of health that men have faced have been concerned with community life, for instance, the control of transmissible disease, the control and improvement of the physical environment (sanitation), the provision of water and food of good quality and in sufficient supply, the provision of medical care, and the relief of disability and destitution. The relative emphasis placed on each of these problems has varied from time to time, but they are all closely related, and from them has come public health as we know it today.

Despite the noted similarities between ancient and contemporary hygiene and sanitation practices, a number of vast differences cannot be ignored. Two of these differences are particularly noteworthy (cf., Rosen, 1958). The first has to do with the reasons behind the practices themselves. Ancient authorities had reasons for implementing hygiene and sanitation measures that differ markedly from those underlying contemporary measures. In ancient times, hygiene and sanitation initiatives were often undertaken for religious as opposed to health reasons. In fact, the belief that "cleanliness is next to godliness" was firmly imbedded in people's psyche in those days. This was the main reason for hygienic behaviour such as bathing and the proper disposal of domestic and other wastes. Egyptians, Mesopotamians, Hebrews and Incas are among the leading ancient cultures that practiced personal and domestic hygiene for religious reasons. The ritual associated with the annual feast known as Citua of the Incas is particularly telling in this connection. During this feast, which took place in September, all members of the Inca society were required to thoroughly clean their bodies, homes and surroundings.

The second difference is related to what was incriminated as the source of the problems that hygiene and sanitation measures were summoned to address. In ancient times health problems were attributed to supernatural forces. In this regard, diseases, especially epidemics, were seen as resulting from divine judgments on the evil deeds of humans. In other words, epidemics were viewed as punishment from the gods. Thus, hygienic behaviour was prescribed as a measure to appease the gods. This disease paradigm and the concomitant prescriptions for dealing with it commanded the health science stage for a very long time. The discovery that disease is a function of environmental factors as opposed to supernatural forces changed thinking in public health for good. This discovery has been dubbed one of the remarkable events in the history of public health and the built environment.

## Public health as an element of town planning

Rather early in the life of public health as a profession, a number of important revelations had been made. One such revelation had to do with pathogenic or filth theory (Herbert, 1999). Based on this theory, many human diseases are a product of gas from decomposing organic matter. From this vantage point, many illnesses are attributable to the air humans breathe. Consequently, human health can be protected through measures designed to ensure clean air. The task of ensuring that air in human settlements was of good quality was assigned to town planning and public health authorities. To appreciate the importance of this task, it is necessary to recall how deplorable living conditions had become during the early phase of the industrial age. It was commonplace to find shoddily constructed workers' residential units attached to, or on the same lot as, factories (Ashton, 1954; 1948). The impetus for maximizing returns on their investments had led unscrupulous real estate investors to subdivide residential units into barely livable space. In some cases, the investors resorted to 'infilling' back gardens, building in courtyards as well as in alleyways and across streets (Njoh, 2007; Herbert, 1999). Most amenities including water and sanitation facilities were shared and typically scant. Usually a whole block was served by no more than a single outdoor latrine and one public water fountain. Very small rooms with little or no ventilation were the order of the day. Given the large family size of the working class of the time, this resulted in excessively overcrowded rooms. Garbage disposal facilities were absent. Consequently, garbage had to be disposed of on the streets or in open fields.

The source of these problems was never in doubt. It was clear to authorities that they were part of the negative externalities of the industrial revolution. Authorities were also quick to realize that addressing the problems required the collaboration of members of different professions and walks of life. In practice most of the responsibility in this regard was shouldered by health professionals, civil engineers and architects-cum-town planners. Therefore, as professions in the form we know them today, public health and town planning emerged to address the health consequences of industrialization. Specifically, the seeds that germinated and blossomed into these twin professions were sowed during the sanitary reform movement. In fact, as I have noted elsewhere, public health and town planning are consanguine relatives with common ancestry in the sanitary movement of the mid-

19th century (Njoh, 2007). "From their birth in the 1800s, town planning and public health, as professions, have always had shared goals" (ibid, 202). Town planning was inspired by the need to protect public health. In Britain, many government bodies were created and placed in charge of different aspects of public health care in the mid-1800s. With the passage of time, British authorities realized the need to deal with the issue of health within a comprehensive as opposed to a piecemeal model. Consequently, about a century later, they established a Ministry of Health in 1919. This action effectively consolidated the medical and public health functions of the British central government under one institutional umbrella.

It is no coincidence that England, industrialization's birthplace also gave birth to the sanitary reform movement. Sanitation and hygiene policy as we know it today was initially promulgated in the mid-1800s. About a century earlier, London had earned the dubious reputation of the industrialized world's most crowded, congested, and disease-ridden city. The city's deplorable conditions had prompted the Reformed Parliament in 1832 to appoint a commission to look into these conditions. The specific task of this commission was to examine the impact of industrialization on the living conditions of the poor.

A radical by the name Edwin Chadwick, who evolved into one of the most dominant sanitary reform figures in Britain, was appointed Assistant to this Commission. He later became its Commissioner, and brought the utilitarian principles of Jeremy Bentham to bear on the Poor Law Inquiry (Rosen, 1858). Most notable of Chadwick's actions, however, was his role in preparing the *Report on the Sanitary Conditions of the Labouring Population of Great Britain* in 1842. This report, as its title suggests, contained disturbing accounts of the conditions of the poor in Britain. Similar perturbing accounts were contained in the works of social critics of the time. Arguably the most forceful of these criticisms appear in Friedrich Engels's classic, *Die Lage der arbeitenden Klasse in England* (i.e., *The Condition of the Working Class in England*). Not long after the release of Engel's work in 1845, British authorities embarked on serious steps to improve living conditions in the country's industrial cities with emphasis on London.

In fact, Britain's landmark health Act of 1848 was enacted only three years subsequent to the release of Engels work. The Act effectively established Britain's Sanitary Law. This and a sister Act of 1875 had the avowed purpose of preventing diseases such as dysentery, typhus, and tuberculosis that result from insalubrious conditions. Apart from acting on the legislative front, British authorities moved to undertake public works projects with the sole purpose of ameliorating health conditions in the industrial towns. In this regard, they constructed elaborate drainage and fresh water supply systems especially in London.

Accounts of sanitation reforms in Britain and Europe in general are often remiss by failing to mention the foresightedness of Edwin Chadwick. Few officials of Chadwick's time matched his zeal in protesting the privatization of public health in general and water in particular. Chadwick, a faithful disciple of Jeremy Bentham, had grown increasingly perturbed by the dominance of *laisez-faire* capitalism in society. With the individualization of the pursuit of wealth, every societal activity had become an acceptable candidate for privatization. Chadwick was bent on ensuring that public health remained a public sector activity. He deployed statistics on urban morbidity and mortality to bolster arguments to the effect that a threat to public health anywhere constituted a threat to public health everywhere (Njoh, 2007). Furthermore, he borrowed generously from the ideas of Bentham. In this regard, he made a strong case for applying the benefits of industrialization towards the greatest good for the greatest numbers. Chadwick's steadfast anti-privatization stance led to the establishment in Britain of instruments of state intervention in the water delivery sector. The creation of the London Metropolitan Water Board exemplifies actions in this regard. The importance of initiatives designed to nationalize water systems such as Chadwick advocated is worth underscoring given that more than a century later, questions relating to whether water should be privatized remain current.

## Eurocentric sanitary and hygiene practices in Africa

The sanitary reforms movement in Britain and Europe in general has contemporary relevance. It is the foundation of most of the sanitation and hygiene measures in vogue throughout contemporary Africa and other parts of the world. In fact, it did not take long for the policies that were developed as part of the sanitary reforms movement in Britain to be adopted in other parts of Europe. However, it took until the official commencement of the European colonial era in Africa (circa, 1884/85) for the policies to be transplanted to Africa. In practice, this meant among other things, the introduction of European notions of building, environmental design, and public health. Here, it is important to note that the philosophy underlying sanitation and hygiene policies in Africa were markedly different from what obtained in Europe. Recall that in Britain, sanitary reformists subscribed to the philosophy of greatest good for the greatest numbers. In Africa, colonial authorities were concerned with protecting exclusively the health of Europeans in the colonies. To be sure, some minimal efforts were made to improve conditions in non-European districts. However, such efforts had two main purposes. The first was to prevent the spread of communicable diseases from these districts to the European enclaves. The other was to facilitate the reproduction of labour for the colonial economy.

Yet, the impact of colonial sanitation and hygiene policies was not, and has never been, limited to Europeans in the colonies. This is particularly because upon the demise of colonialism, the policies were inherited wholesale by indigenous authorities. One of the most impactful of these policies is articulated in the form of building codes. Building codes derive their importance in public health mainly from the fact that they serve as instruments for regulating the development of physical structures in the built environment. The importance of building codes, and the concomitant regulations and standards in the context of this book is grounded in their implications for questions of sustainability. To be sustainable, the codes, regulations and standards have to be contextual. However, because they were transplanted from settings that are completely different in economic, social and cultural terms, from Africa, they are not. To shed further light on this point, it is necessary to consider the meaning of the related terms, regulations, codes and standards. The meaning proffered in the report of the UN Seminar of Experts on Building Codes and Regulations in Developing Countries held in Tallberg and Stockholm, Sweden some three decades ago is apt (see UNCHS, 1980).

Regulations are a product of legal actions. In other words, they are legal instruments that must be enforced through designated national and/or local channels. Such channels typically include agencies of national and local governmental bodies. In terms of their raison d'être, building regulations are designed to influence all activities with respect to the built environment. These regulations derive their legitimacy from the belief that they are necessary as a means of ensuring the public good. Therefore, Africa's contemporary building codes, most of which are a legacy of the colonial past, can be considered to be neither sustainable nor legitimate. This is because they were crafted for a completely different setting, and never intended to protect the health and safety of the general public.

Building codes have as their avowed purpose, the promotion of public health, safety and welfare of a building's occupants in particular and the public in general. They are typically of two varieties, namely specification-oriented and performance-based. The former stipulate the exact type of materials to be used in completing specific elements of a building. Performance-based codes specify the standard to be met by any given building element, and allow the builder or architect to select the necessary material. Building codes also stipulate requirements for the use and occupancy of buildings. This aspect of building codes has a direct bearing on questions of health, hazards, and safety. Building codes are further concerned with structural design, and amenities such as plumbing. Again, because building codes in Africa are a colonial legacy, their sustainability is questionable. Yet, if carefully thought-out, building codes can be used to promote not only public health but also national economic development.

Hardly any aspect of building and environmental control has as much relevance to the discourse on sustainability as standards. This is because standards, more than any other aspect of this control are most affected by location, socio-cultural context and prevailing economic conditions (cf., UNCHS, 1981). The standards that resulted from the sanitary reform initiatives of the 19th century in England, and later the rest of Europe, regulated building and spatial design. In this regard, the standards stipulated aspects of building and environmental design such as room sizes, distances between buildings, the sizes of windows, thickness of walls, the slope of roofs, and so on. In addition, they enacted measures to achieve important values such as privacy, comfort and convenience. There is certainly no question that these items and values are location-bound and culturally relative. Thus, the fact that they were designed for Europe and transplanted to Africa renders their appropriateness and sustainability highly questionable.

## Colonialism and the public health problematic in Africa

As noted earlier, since the late-20th century, public health and town planning have largely drifted apart. As Corburn (2004: 541) observed, "although public health and urban planning emerged with the common goal of preventing urban outbreaks of infectious diseases, there is little overlap between the fields today." A major shift in thinking about disease etiology occurred in Europe at the twilight of the colonial era in Africa in the late-19th century when miasma ceded its place to germ theory. Germ theory attributed infectious diseases to specific agents, particularly microbes. The shift in thinking about diseases resulted in public health professionals withdrawing from activities designed to improve urban physical structures. Thenceforth, health professionals re-channeled their energy into laboratory research designed to better understand microbes as well as device measures such as vaccines capable of inoculating human populations against infectious diseases. Thus, the shift in thinking about disease that occurred in the late-19th century resulted in moving public health from the human physical environment into the laboratory. On their part, planners came to see themselves as professionally unqualified to conceive, formulate and even implement health policies. Several decades subsequent to these developments in Europe and North America, their reverberations are currently being felt in Africa. Consequently, post-colonial administrative reforms in countries throughout the continent have strived to separate the functions of public health, which were typically under the same government ministerial body as town planning during the colonial era and the early post-colonial era.

At that time, public health elements featured prominently in town planning legislation. In fact, town planning practice was pre-occupied with implementing health policy. For instance, legislation and codes requiring ample ventilation for buildings were widespread in colonial cities throughout Africa (Njoh, 2007). Similarly commonplace were town planning ordinances designed to control urban design, layouts and morphological relationships between streets, blocks and dwelling units. It is important to note that despite the readiness of colonial authorities to transplant these and cognate pieces of legislation to Africa, they were enacted with European towns and municipalities in mind. Yet, it is clear that at the onset of the Industrial Revolution, Europe faced health problems that were markedly different from those that plagued Africa during the colonial period, and continue to menace the continent today. How have these received pieces of legislation affected and continue to affect spatial structures in Africa? What are their implications for the socio-economic development aspirations of African countries?

The bifurcation of the responsibilities of town planners and public health officials has happened throughout Africa. In most countries on the continent, officials from the two fields typically work under separate ministerial bodies, and collaboration between them is usually rare. Hygiene and sanitation infrastructure have become secondary on the priority ladder of health professionals. A related development has been a relegation of the health implications of the built environment to a tertiary position in the discourse on public health. However, I hasten to note that these developments have been documented exclusively in the developed world (see e.g., Coburn, 2004).

Studies of developments in the field of hygiene, sanitation and public health in the developing world, let alone Africa, remain scant. Also worthy of note is the fact that government policies in most African countries have typically failed to recognize public health and urban planning as the inextricably intertwined entities that they are. Rather, for reasons hinted at above, the two have operated in isolation. In this regard, urban planning has focused exclusively on the form of built space, while matters of hygiene and sanitation have been viewed as falling under the purview of public health officials. This partially explains the fact that most African countries are not on track to meet the hygiene-and-sanitation-related targets of the Millennium Development Goals (MDGs).

However, it is necessary to caution against the danger of overgeneralization here. There is a tendency in development discourse to lump all African countries into one category. This is erroneous, especially with respect to matters of hygiene and sanitation. To be sure, African countries differ markedly in this regard. Hygiene and sanitation conditions are better in some of the countries than in others. Stated alternatively, some African countries have made more progress than others in efforts to address the hygiene and sanitation needs of their inhabitants. In fact, progress reports by units of the United Nations, such as the WHO/UNICEF's Joint Monitoring Programme (JMP), lend credence to this assertion. However, the relevant literature contains no explanation for this phenomenon. An important objective of this book is to redress this deficiency in the literature.

## Some preliminary questions and hypotheses

I posit two main interrelated factors as determinants of hygiene and sanitation policies and the resultant conditions in Africa. Both factors are rooted in European colonial urban planning and spatial development policies. The first is the ideology of race upon which health policies in the built environment in colonial Africa were based. The second is the tendency on the part of the indigenous leadership in Africa to adhere to inherited colonial spatial development policies. This implies unwillingness on the part of the leadership to develop innovative development policies in concert with contemporary dynamics. The book shows how these policies have served to aggravate, rather than improve, public health conditions. Understanding the link between these misguided policies and the hygiene and sanitation problematic in Africa is not only of academic importance. Rather, such an understanding holds immense promise for domestic and international policy makers concerned with improving health conditions on the continent. Knowledge of the implications of past policies on public health can help contemporary and future policy makers avoid repeating the mistakes of their predecessors.

Of particular concern are policies that sought to, or effectively, alter the built environment with the avowed aim of improving public health. The avowed aims of the policies notwithstanding, they have been driven mostly by ideology and the need to accomplish other objectives of the colonial or post-colonial state. Thus, the policies are not generated by a genuine concern for the welfare of the citizenry. Before sketching the plan of this book, I present a vivid picture of the history of modern town planning, especially as a tool for promoting and protecting public health in modern Africa.

In more recent history, European imperial authorities recorded evidence of a concern for public health such as wells and pit latrines in human settlements prior to the formal onset of colonialism on the continent (Bigon, 2005). In fact, despite the barrage of negative myths about deplorable sanitary conditions in Africa, some have uncovered evidence suggesting that these conditions were comparable to those of human settlements in the West (see e.g., Brown, 1994). Thus, the frequent disparaging characterization of health conditions on the continent by Europeans was therefore unwarranted. Here, it is worth noting that the same health problems, particularly epidemics such as the bubonic plague, tuberculosis, and cholera had wreaked as much havoc on France and Britain in the 1830s, as they did on Africa.

However, it is necessary to note that the methods that had been adopted to respond to these epidemics and other health problems were not universal. Rather, the methods and strategies drew inspiration from the proximate environment and concomitant culture. As noted earlier, it was not until the colonial era that sanitary and health policies were transplanted wholesale from Europe to Africa. Thus, the roots of public health as an objective of spatial and physical development policy in contemporary Africa are traceable to Europe. Recall that the policies are derivatives of the health acts that were promulgated to address the negative externalities of the industrial revolution in Europe.

European colonial authorities were obsessively pre-occupied with efforts to alter and/or control the spatial structure of human settlements throughout Africa. Several reasons were advanced to justify these efforts. However, none of the reasons was as frequently invoked as the need to promote public health in the colonial territories. To be sure, the European town planning movement from which modern town planning in Africa drew its inspiration did not emerge specifically to deal with problems of public health. However, by the onset of the European colonial era in Africa, the need to promote public health had become a preoccupation of town planning. With the advent of the industrial revolution, health concerns rapidly moved to the front and center of town planning in Europe.

The colonial era in Africa coincided with the afore-described developments in Europe. Hence, the town planning model that colonial authorities introduced in Africa had as its foremost objective the promotion and protection of human health. However, as I have observed before, colonial 'public health' schemes sought to promote and protect exclusively the health of Europeans. Thus, the authorities had a rather twisted definition of the term 'public' as it was anything but inclusive. That is a whole different matter. Of essence here is the fact that public health was treated as an integral part of spatial planning. Yet, it is doubtful that without Edwin Chadwick modernist town planning in Africa or elsewhere for that matter would have contained public health elements. Recall that Chadwick had methodically deployed empirical data to demonstrate that the Industrial Revolution and accompanying urbanization had serious health consequences. Also recall that he was able to persuasively argue against privatizing public health. The establishment of public health as a government function in colonial Africa is attributable, at least in part, to Chadwick's actions.

These and similar questions are yet to be adequately addressed despite the fact that a few major works (e.g., Home, 1997; King, 1990; Simon, 1992; Njoh, 2007), and several scholarly articles (e.g., Abu-Lughod, 1965; Chokor, 1993; Njoh, 2002) have examined the process by which European planning models were transplanted to Africa. Almost completely absent from the literature are works seeking to promote understanding of the relationship between public health and town planning on the continent. Thus, there is a gulf in the relevant literature. This gulf concerns the implications for spatial, social and economic development of public health elements of town planning. The main purpose of this book is to contribute to efforts addressed to closing this gap. The book accomplishes its avowed task by attempting to address the following five questions.

1. What is the historical and contemporary relationship between modernist planning and public health in Africa?
2. How have public health elements of modernist planning affected the form (i.e., spatial structure) and function (i.e., effectiveness) of the built environment in Africa?
3. What is the role of ideology in shaping urban public health elements of town planning in Africa?
4. What is the current state of hygiene and sanitation in Africa?
5. What sustainable steps can be taken to improve hygiene and sanitation conditions in Africa?

The importance of these questions is amplified by the fact that urban public health impacts not only national development but also socio-economic development and human wellbeing. In his address to the New York Academy of Medicine under the caption, "Global Health: Challenges, Capacity and Responsibility" on May 9, 2006, the Secretary-General of the United Nations at the time, Kofi Annan, underscored the importance of urban public health, especially in developing countries, when he made the following statement (Annan, on-line, para. 22).

> We must dispel the notion that public health challenges are simply public health issues. Major health challenges are also development issues and sometimes security issues. So, our response must engage the highest levels of government, civil society, business and finance. We must abandon traditional bureaucratic thinking and work across ministries and departments to forge a holistic approach.

Today, more than half of humankind lives in cities. That is more than 3 billion people. Nearly one billion or one in every six human beings is an urban slum dweller living without adequate shelter and basic services. This figure is expected to rise to 2 billion over the next 25 years. As poverty grows increasingly urban, the greatest impact will be felt in the very poorest countries. Urban poverty, in turn, creates an entry point for disease and ill health. Millions of people are homeless. The most vulnerable, including women and children, are the first victims of violence, crime, overcrowding and all the health hazards associated with inhuman living conditions in rapidly growing cities. It is in these urban killing fields that epidemics take their heaviest toll.

A significant portion of the book is pre-occupied with one specific aspect of public health, namely hygiene and sanitation. The importance of this aspect of public health has been recognized at the international level especially since the last decade. As a testament to this recognition, hygiene and sanitation were added to the list of the Millennium Development Goals (MDGs). We hasten to note that the MDGs were initially established by the United Nations Development Programme (UNDP) in 2000. Further testament to the acknowledgement of sanitation as a critical objective of development can be gleaned from two sources. First, the UNDP's Human Development Report for 2006 featured water and sanitation as an issue deserving of urgent international attention. Second, the year 2008 was anointed as the International Year of Sanitation (IYS).

Despite its attentiveness to the critical health issues of the day, the book has a very modest objective. It seeks at one level to promote understanding of the nature of the relationship between urban public health and town planning in Africa. Here, the intention is to identify and discuss specific public policies that have served to aggravate rather than improve health conditions in Africa. At another level, the book strives to shed some light on the nature of one specific aspect of Africa's public health problematic, namely hygiene and sanitation. Initially, the focus is on the colonial era. Of particular interest are the magnitude and complexity of the continent's hygiene and sanitation problem. Also of interest are the factors that have contributed to complicating efforts geared towards arresting the problem. The passages that follow are dedicated to outlining the book's content.

**Plan of the book**

Chapter 2 follows this introductory chapter. It begins the journey into exploring public health elements of spatial policies by analyzing the role of ideology in shaping these elements. A substantial part of the chapter focuses on hygiene and sanitation legislation in pre-colonial Africa. Popular belief holds that European colonial authorities introduced hygiene and sanitation elements of spatial design in Africa. This is erroneous. The truth is that such elements constituted part of spatial planning policies during the pre-colonial era. In fact, planned and systematic steps designed to improve the health of residents of large human settlements not only pre-dated colonialism but the presence of Europeans in Africa. What was the nature of the health problems of large human settlements in pre-colonial Africa? What steps were taken to address these problems? The chapter initially highlights the indigenous origins of public health policies in pre-colonial Africa. Then, it examines colonial and post-colonial hygiene and sanitation initiatives in the context of spatial development.

Chapter 3 focuses on public health within the broader context of the European colonial project in Africa. An important objective of the chapter is to depict the health components of colonial urban planning. Initially, the chapter retraces the common roots of urban planning and public health to the industrial revolution. Then, it shows how colonial authorities employed concern for the health and wellbeing of Europeans as a pretext to racially segregate spatial structures throughout Africa.

Chapter 4 takes a further look at the issue of race, which appeared to have been the basis for most spatially-tied health policies in colonial Africa. In particular, the chapter shows how the race ideology that was in vogue at the time constituted the basis for racial residential segregation as a prophylaxis against malaria. The relevant literature subscribes to the notion that European colonial segregation policies were informed by the limited knowledge of tropical diseases of the time. Within this frame of thinking, racism had nothing to do with these policies. The chapter advances an alternate viewpoint. It is argued that such policies were simply an embodiment and reflection of the racist thinking of the time. Public health as a rationale for racial segregation, the chapter argues, was therefore duplicitous.

With the demise of colonialism more than half a century ago, one would have expected more novel urban planning policies in Africa. This is not the case. Rather, the indigenous leadership resorted to inheriting, sharpening and implementing the planning policies of their departing colonial predecessors. These policies, which commonly go under the name, modernist planning, remain in vogue throughout the continent. What are the implications of this for public health promotion initiatives on the continent? The main objective of Chapter 5 is to tackle this question. More importantly, the chapter takes a closer look at the health elements of modern town planning with a view to promoting understanding of their nature, strengths and weaknesses in efforts to wrestle with the myriad public health problems prevalent in urban areas throughout the continent. As stated earlier, the roots of public health elements of modern town planning on the continent are traceable to Europe. European colonial authorities introduced these elements simultaneously with modernist town planning. The fact that European colonial authorities transplanted modern town planning to Africa is fairly well-known. What is however, contentious or little known is why transplanting modern town planning schemes with their concomitant European cultural baggage was deemed a necessary part of the colonial project. Why did European colonial authorities transplant modern town planning schemes, particularly the health elements of these schemes to Africa? The chapter also wrestles with this question. It further identifies and discusses on the one hand, the many ways in which the implementation of the stated elements shape urban form and function. On the other hand, it shows how the elements are, or ought to be, affected by urban form.

Agents of development have long recognized that the spatial structures that were introduced by European colonial authorities in Africa are antithetical to socio-economic development efforts on the continent. However, the fact that these structures have negative implications for efforts to promote and protect public health has received hardly any attention. Yet, it is obvious that efforts to institutionalize non-motorized modes of transportation as part of a broader strategy to encourage people to indulge in passive physical exercise are likely to be unsuccessful. One reason for this, as I have noted elsewhere is that schemes designed to compartmentalize land use activities as part of the efforts by colonial authorities to promote spatial order often resulted in unnecessarily elongating the distance between residential areas and workplaces (Njoh, 1999; 1995). In some cases, the the work places such as office parks were/are located at the top of hills while residential areas were/are located at the foot of these hills. What are the health implications of such spatial structures for public health? This question is at the heart of the discussion in Chapter 5.

The next three chapters of the book focus on the current state of hygiene and sanitation on the continent. Hygiene and sanitation are seen to encompass three broad components as described in Table 1.1. The schema developed by the United Nations Children's Fund (UNICEF), which divides the continent into three sub-regions is adopted. The three sub-regions include the West and Central Africa Region (Chapter 6), the Eastern and Southern Africa Region (Chapter 7), and the Northern Africa Region (Chapter 8). Each of these sub-regions is examined with a view to: 1) assessing prevailing hygiene and sanitation conditions therein, and 2) its progress towards meeting the relevant target of the Millennium Development Goals (MDGs).

**Table 1.1 Main components of hygiene and sanitation**

| | |
|---|---|
| Sanitation | Safe collection, storage, treatment and disposal/re-use/ recycling of human excreta (faeces and urine); Management,/re-use/recycling of solid waste (rubbish); Collection and management of industrial waste products (including hospital wastes, chemical/radio-active and other dangerous substances). |
| Hygiene | Safe water storage; Safe hand-washing; Safe treatment of foodstuffs. |
| Water Management | Drainage and disposal/re-use/recycling of household waste water (also referred to as 'grey water'); Drainage of storm water; Treatment and disposal/re-use/recycling of sewage effluents. |

*Source*: Tearfund (2007).

The sub-regional case studies point to significant disparities with respect to access to improved hygiene and sanitation facilities at the international and inter-regional levels. What factors account for these disparities? Certainly, these factors are plentiful and obviously complex. However, within the framework of this book, it is hypothesized that colonialism accounts for a substantial portion of the disparities. Chapter 9 takes on the task of testing this hypothesis. Thus, the chapter takes the discussion to a different level. It attempts to quantify the connection between colonial experience and development operationalized in terms of access to improved hygiene and sanitation. Accordingly, it posits access to water and sanitation services and facilities—two important components of public health—as a function of colonial experience.

Chapter 10 constitutes the final chapter of the book. An important objective of the chapter is to determine why, despite the attention accorded urban public health in Africa, the problem remains nagging and seemingly intractable. To be sure, a plethora of factors account for this nightmarish situation. However, there has been a tendency to rely exclusively on borrowed remedies while ignoring indigenous knowledge. There has also been a propensity towards attributing the problem to a lack of financial and other tangible resources. In contrast, the chapter advocates indigenous knowledge and the need to incorporate citizen participation as potentially sustainable strategies to deal with the situation.

**Target audience of the book**

Urban planners, public health officials and international entities involved in promoting development in the built environment in Africa will find a lot of grist for their mills in this book. Another group that will find utility in this book are students of the history and political economy of Africa. In addition, academics involved in research and teaching on development in Africa will benefit enormously from the material in the book. In this regard, the book can be used either for reference purposes or as a secondary textbook in senior undergraduate or graduate courses on development planning and administration, global public health, as well as sustainable development. Finally, members of the general public with more than a passing interest in urban public health, urban development and socio-economic development in Africa will find utility in this book.

# Chapter 2
# The State, Ideology, Health and Built Space in Africa

## Introduction

Many would agree that urban planning as an instrument of public health has failed to register significant positive results in Africa. In fact, it is arguable that urban planning policies have actually contributed to aggravating public health problems on the continent. Why is this the case? Consensus is lacking as far as answers to this question go. There is a tendency to attribute development failures such as these exclusively to the lack of financial resources. This chapter deviates from the norm. It puts forth alternative explanations for the inability of urban planning to deliver on its promise to promote and protect public health. It attributes the failure of planning in this connection to three major factors (cf., Njoh, 2008). These include: 1) the nature and behaviour of the state, 2) the out of context nature of health policies, and 3) the fact that health policies are driven by ideology as opposed to science. The chapter has a secondary purpose, namely to provide a conceptual foundation for discussions in subsequent chapters. It begins by exploring the concept of ideology. Then, it delves into the institutional and administrative problems that have historically bedevilled public health initiatives in Africa.

## Ideology, urban planning and public health in Africa

The term ideology can be appreciated at three different but overlapping levels. At the first level, ideology can be taken to constitute a body of ideas that are designed to realize certain goals of powerful groups, classes or individuals within society. To the extent that urban planning is a function of the state, it is informative to appreciate the concept of ideology within a Marxian framework. Within this framework, the state is seen not as a fair-minded arbiter of change in society. Rather, it is viewed as a tool of dominant societal groups. From this vantage point, it is easy to appreciate the importance of ideology, particularly when the concept is taken to connote the use of false pretexts to camouflage the true intentions of a governing body.

At the second level, ideology embodies two distinct conceptual categories—the 'particular' and the 'total' (Mannheim, 1985). The particular conception of ideology is implied when the term denotes the scepticism that citizens, especially marginalized groups, harbour with respect to the ideas, doctrines and actions of dominant groups and individuals (Njoh, 2008). Third, ideology can be seen as comprising the normative goals of society and the organizational structures, methods, techniques and principles that are adopted to achieve these goals.

Ideology is at the root of development policies in general and public health elements of town planning in particular. Here, it is necessary to draw attention to the fact that planning itself qualifies as an ideology. This is especially because of its professed (ideological) goals. As Donald Foley (1960) has noted, the following constitute some of the most prominent of these goals:

- Reconciling competing claims for the use of limited land in order to provide a consistent, balanced and orderly arrangement of land uses;
- Providing a physical environment capable of promoting a healthy and civilized lifestyle; and
- Providing the physical basis for a better community life, and striving toward the provision of low-density residential areas, and fostering local livelihood as well as controlling urban growth.

Other ideological goals that have been enunciated by especially modernist planning initiatives include ensuring:

1. the development of a functional, safe and healthy built environment;
2. the development of an aesthetically pleasing urban environment;
3. the harmonious growth and development of urban areas and regions; and
4. the formulation and implementation of policies to promote sustainable urban development.

These and cognate ideological goals have constituted the avowed aims of urban planning in Africa since the colonial era. In practice, authorities tend to take actions that deviate from, and sometimes, contradict, these goals. This is because, as agents of the state, the primary duty of planning authorities is to protect the state's interests at any given moment. This was the case during the colonial era. The situation remains unchanged today, half a century following the demise of colonialism. The reason for this can be better understood with knowledge of the state in modern Africa as contrasted with its pre-colonial predecessor.

### Pre-Colonial Africa

It is not uncommon to come across analyses of the political economy of Africa that credit European colonialism with the introduction of statehood as a form of political organization on the continent. Jeffrey Herbst (2000) is among the few scholars who have acknowledged the existence of states and state systems predating the European colonial era in Africa. He has lambasted the unimaginative characterization of pre-colonial Africa as a stateless society. As Herbst noted, some have gone so far as to describe pre-colonial Africa as "a continental archipelago of loosely defined political systems" (Herbst, 2005: 36). Yet, pre-colonial Africa was in many ways, similar to medieval Europe. Recall that in medieval Europe the church and other societal entities shared sovereignty. An identical situation was in vogue in pre-colonial Africa. African states of that time were complete with a constitution and administrative institutions organized along functional lines. One case in point is the Fanti Confederation in present-day Ghana. In 1871, and after having just emerged victorious in a war with its neighbours, the Confederation moved swiftly to adopt a constitution, and to craft a national development plan. The plan contained detailed information on different aspects of development including road and other infrastructure building projects. Such details included the specific width of the roads and the surfacing materials to be used. Section 26 of the Constitution stipulated that the roads had to be fifteen feet (or five meters) wide (Herbst, 2005: 42). The relevance of road widths to public health and safety is easy to appreciate. Wider roadways tend to be significantly safer than narrow ones. This suggests that public health was an element of urban and regional planning in Africa as far back as the pre-colonial era. Also, as I have noted elsewhere, ideology was at the root of most of these elements (see Njoh, 2009). In fact, as noted in Chapter 1, urban planning, dating back to antiquity, has always incorporated elements of public health. Efforts to shape the built environment would be non-existent in the absence of a need to improve public health. This point is well-established. What is far less known, and likely to be the subject of rancorous debate, ancient and pre-colonial planning in Africa was also driven by ideology. Conceivably, health elements of spatial planning in pre-colonial Africa were influenced by some aspects of indigenous tradition that could be considered ideological.

Knowledge of pre-colonial planning and health practices and institutions in Africa hold enormous promise for contemporary efforts to improve living conditions on the continent. The value of traditional socio-cultural, economic and political institutions in the health domain is increasingly acknowledged. A recent report by the Economic Commission for Africa (ECA), appropriately entitled, *Relevance of African Traditional Institutions of Governance* underscored the potentially valuable role that traditional institutions can play in sensitizing the population on health issues such as HIV/AIDS (ECA, 2007: v).

To be sure, the traditional institutions in question were created and led by indigenous authorities. The authorities were also responsible for conceiving, formulating and enacting public policies, including those governing public health practices and institutions. As societal elites, these authorities viewed themselves as responsible for ensuring the welfare of the general public. With this belief, and conceivably influenced by their own world view, they proceeded to enact public health and spatial policies. Thus, it is safe to say that health elements of spatial policy in pre-colonial Africa were influenced by indigenous elitism.

Researchers have largely ignored the fact that so-called primitive planning contained these elements, which were stipulated based on indigenous knowledge. Yet, throughout Africa, from Dakar to Mogadishu, and from Cairo to Cape Town, evidence attesting to the existence of activities designed to protect and/or promote the health status of the general public before the European conquest abounds (see e.g., Waite, 1987; Njoh, 2006). To say that the elements were driven by indigenous elitism is to acknowledge the fact they were the products of the knowledge, proclivities and vision of the indigenous ruling elites. Here, it is important to note that what these elites considered to be the general good of the community at large, that is, the 'public welfare' may not have necessarily coincided with the views of members of that so-called 'general public.'

Concern for public health in pre-colonial Africa grew as hamlets evolved into villages. For a while, these villages were small and widely dispersed. However, with the passage of time, they grew demographically and geographically. Concomitant with this growth was a rise in density levels and a proliferation of health problems. As socio-political organizations, pre-colonial African villages were headed by lineage heads. These lineage heads were in some cases under the jurisdiction of senior lineage heads or clan heads and minor chiefs (Njoh, 2009). Minor chiefs had control over several villages and/or clans. They were responsible for addressing many issues relating to the welfare of members of their clans and/ or villages. The measures that were adopted to address these issues were not systematic. Also, they did not carry much force. The necessary force for enforcing or implementing the measures was never known until about the tenth century. This is when a plethora of kingdoms began emerging throughout the continent. This period also marks the emergence of statehood as a form of political organization in Africa. Thus, contrary to popular belief, well organized and highly centralized political structures that bore hallmarks of modern states pre-dated the arrival of Europeans on the continent (Njoh, 2006; Herbst, 2000). With the emergence of such structures, particularly kingdoms, the ruling elites assumed responsibility over all matters of a public nature. Health problems fell under two categories. Small health matters were placed under the jurisdiction of family heads. Larger health issues, such as those affecting whole villages, fell under the auspices of the ruling elites such as priests, chiefs or kings.

Larger health issues necessitated intervention by ruling elites. Examples of these issues include: hygiene and sanitation, epidemics, environmental degradation, draughts, food shortages, and sorcery-induced ailments. The upkeep, particularly in terms of hygiene and sanitation, of public places, including market squares, the chief's/king's courtyard, springs and other potable water sources, and rivers were the responsibility of all members of the community. The ruling authorities typically set aside a specific day of the week or month on which every member of the community was required to participate in the cleaning and upkeep of these places and/or facilities. On such days, people were divided into teams and assigned specific tasks. Such tasks included, preparing the food that would be consumed at the end of the day.

The strategies that were employed to deal with other health problems varied based on the nature of the problem. According to traditional Africans, diseases and other health problems are generated by spirits, which are in turn tied to ancestry. Ancestry can be divided into two sub-groups (Waite, 1987). The one is tied to founders of the individual family. The other is linked to the founders of the community. Health problems such as the aforementioned belong to this second group of spirits, which are also known as territorial or tutelary spirits. Societal elites controlled the propitiation of spirits of this second order on behalf of the community at large.

In the event of an epidemic outbreak, authorities took serious steps with spatial implications (Waite, 1987). Examples of such steps include, limiting the movement of people, prohibiting conjugal relationships and congregation in public places. Other examples include prohibiting people from engaging in otherwise everyday activities such as house-to-house visitations. It was taboo in most societies in traditional Africa to defecate or dump in lakes, rivers or any body of water for that matter. Concern with environmental pollution led the ruling elite to issue edicts that further treated such behaviour as criminal. In the ancient Kingdom of Ashanti, for instance, a unit of local government under the Public Works Department was assigned the sole function of enforcing laws designed to maintain proper hygiene and sanitation standards (Njoh, 2006). Citizens were required to collect and burn, in designated locations, all rubbish and offal from their homes every morning.

Apart from more obvious concerns such as those catalogued above, pre-colonial Africans also lumped under the rubric of public health, acts of God. Prominent in this regard were natural disasters such as draughts and resultant food shortages. A common approach to dealing with this problem was to summon priests, chiefs, kings and other community leaders. These leaders would in turn, summon rainmakers to invoke the ancestral spirits, and pray through them to the Almighty God to provide rain. People were required to settle in fertile crescents and valleys, where they could farm. This prevented any possibility of starvation and related problems.

Finally, there is the matter of sorcery-induced ailments. Sorcery, which involves anti-social and nefarious acts, was a serious public health issue in pre-colonial Africa. To appreciate sorcery's public health status, one must first understand the fact that sorcery was incriminated as the cause of several sudden deaths in pre-colonial Africa. Particularly because sorcery accusations were made in public, sorcery was considered to fall under the public as opposed to the family domain. Accordingly, as in other matters of public or communal importance, the ruling elites intervened to minimize possible damage to the community at large. It is necessary to note that with the emergence of the ideology of modernization during the colonial era, public accusations of sorcery and concomitant activities were actively discouraged (Waite, 1987).

## Colonial Africa

The conceptual meaning of the term 'state' remains a subject of fierce debate. Even more heated is the debate on how to characterize and interpret the nature, significance and role of the state in society. For the purpose of the present discussion, the major characterizations and interpretations of the state are classified into three different but overlapping schools of thought, namely liberal pluralists, Marxists and neo-Weberians (Njoh, 2003; Njoh, 1999; Glassman and Samatar, 1997).

Based on the Liberal pluralist school, the state is a fair-minded arbiter of social change. In this capacity, the actions of the state in society are not meant to protect the interest of any specific group. Rather, its actions are designed to protect the interest of society at large. Additionally, the state exists to preside over disputes amongst societal groups while ensuring the attainment of societal goals (Muir, 1997; Glassman and Samatar, 1997; Johnston, 1982). Within the framework of liberal pluralist theories, the state is seen ideally as a neutral entity that is free from corruption and influence from powerful and dominant societal groups. From a more practical perspective, influence on the state cannot be avoided. However, at least in theory, every individual in society, through membership in social groups can successfully influence the actions of the state, especially at the decision making stage. Unfortunately, where access to the levers of power is the exclusive preserve of a few, the ordinary citizen has no realistic chance of influencing the state's actions. In the colonial situation, as shown below, the state existed at the pleasure of, and to serve the interest of, the colonizer. From a Marxist perspective, it would be erroneous to characterize the state as a fair-minded arbiter of social change.

Marxists and neo-Marxists see the state as anything but a neutral umpire in societal matters. Rather, they see the state as "an expression of broader patterns of domination and exploitation within society" (Glassman and Samatar, 1997: 166). From this vantage point, the state's actions must be judged in light of, first and foremost, its own interests. These interests are more often than not, an embodiment and reflection of the interests of dominant societal groups or classes. Writing as far back as 1848, Karl Marx had suggested that "the executive of the modern state is but a committee for managing the common affairs of the whole bourgeoisie" (quoted in Njoh, 1999: 112; Muir, 1997: 83). Ralph Miliband (1969: 5) later echoed Marx's sentiment by stating that the state is nothing but "the coercive instrument of the ruling class."

Neo-Weberian conceptualizations of the state differ from Marxist and Neo-Marxist versions in one fundamental way. They accord little importance to the explanatory power of economic forces (Mann, 1988; Giddens, 1985). Neo-Weberians tend to concentrate on the formal institutions and agents jointly comprising the rather nebulous entity called the state. The analytic foci of scholars of this persuasion are usually, but not always, the motives of these institutions. For neo-Weberians, economic forces are less powerful than the specific mechanisms, instruments and structures of the state, as predictors of social outcomes.

The state in colonial Africa was peculiar. Its peculiarity is noteworthy when one considers the fact that it lacked most of the attributes of the modern state. If at all the colonial state qualified as a state it is thanks to the following four reasons (Young, 1994). First, it controlled territory, albeit vaguely defined. Second, it had a population of people under its auspices. Third, it was sovereign, had enormous power, and possessed a set of laws. Finally, it was an actor in the international arena.

Another peculiarity of the colonial state worth noting is the fact that it was incapable of exercising the major imperatives of a modern republican state. These imperatives include hegemony, autonomy, security, legitimacy, revenue, and accumulation. The peculiarity of the colonial state has been attributed to a number of factors, three of which are worth mentioning here. These factors include the following (Chazan et al., 1992). First, the state in colonial Africa was established at a time when both the modern metropolitan and the generic colonial state had already been created. Consequently, there was no room for experimentation. Second, the colonial state in Africa came into being through conquest. As a result, it boasted a hegemony that was excessively coercive and forcefully imposed. Other notable attributes of this state are that, it lacked legitimacy, controlled territories with vague geographic boundaries, and possessed an exceedingly weak revenue base. This last point deserves elaboration. The paltry budget of the colonial state thwarted any attempt to address the myriad health or other problems that characterized the colonized territories. The decision to target exclusively European enclaves for health and other public infrastructure development projects was probably a function of budgetary constraint. Colonial governments throughout Africa faced this problem. Another problem that colonial states in Africa encountered had to do with sovereignty. Strictly speaking, colonial states were never sovereign. In truth, the states were controlled from the colonial master nation. Therefore, they possessed hardly any powers of their own.

The foregoing characteristics of the state in colonial Africa had far-reaching implications for health policymaking in the colonies. Colonial officials on the ground frequently disagreed with their bosses in the metropolitan country over necessary policy actions in the colonies. In almost all cases, the directives of colonial bosses in the colonial master nation tromped the recommendations of officials in the colonies. One case in point relates to the decision to adopt racial segregation as a strategy to combat the malaria epidemic in colonial Nigeria. MacGregor, a medical doctor by training, and at the time the Governor of the colony, was against racial residential segregation. He believed segregation could not serve as a prophylaxis against malaria. However, he was overruled by Joseph Chamberlain, the British Colonial Secretary. Regardless of its therapeutic value, Chamberlain was bent on making segregation the official policy in all British colonies in tropical Africa.

The resource problem of colonial governments is succinctly captured by Liora Bigon in her discussion of the British colonial experience in West Africa. "In British West Africa, conquest and administration were only backed by meagre resources, run on shoestring budgets and chronically underfunded and undermanned" (Bigon, 2005: 249). Their paltry budgets notwithstanding, colonial governments in Africa were charged with many onerous tasks. Prominent among these tasks were the consolidation of colonial rule, the maintenance of ties with colonial master nations, and the promotion of colonial capitalism. Capitalist motives ensured that only projects with obvious and verifiable economic benefits could be implemented. Thus, it is easy to appreciate the fact that the health needs of most Africans hardly ever appeared in the colonial government healthcare budget. In fact, only the few Africans who served in limited capacities in the colonial government were allowed access to the healthcare services of colonial governments. The fact that colonial governments operated on shoestring budgets also explains the frequent use of military personnel in the colonial civil service. Military personnel were common especially in the French colonies.

The imperatives of colonial governance compelled what were effectively weak and fragile states in Africa to develop an interventionist and authoritarian proclivity. Yet another shared attribute of states in colonial Africa, irrespective of their ideological inclinations, is the fact that they justified their existence on the grounds of attaining the ideological goals of civilization and pacification. The policies that were enacted and/or implemented throughout colonial Africa must be evaluated with this in mind. Such policies, including those whose avowed aim was to improve public health were designed to actually attain these goals.

Colonial governments were set up to serve as custodians of the resources of the colonized territories. These governments were under strict orders to ensure the collection and onward transmission of these resources to the colonial master nations. At the same time, they were expected to safeguard the social and economic interests of all Europeans based in the colonies. Health ranked high among these interests especially because of the disease-ridden nature of Africa. Colonial governments throughout the region were directed to implement a litany of policies in this regard. One policy with spatial implications in this connection was the location of exclusive European enclaves on high altitudes that were airy and well drained. These attributes were believed to be capable of improving human health based on the disease theory of miasma that was in vogue at the time. Conversely, Africans were confined to unhealthy locales such as swamps, ravines and creeks.

As stated above, protecting the economic interest of Europeans constituted another responsibility of the colonial state. The need to protect this interest necessitated the promotion of the capitalist mode of production. In practice, this entailed minimization of overhead costs in order to maximize profits. Accordingly, as far as public health went, the colonial state spent only as little as was necessary to prevent epidemic outbreaks. Such outbreaks were often dreaded because of their ability to hinder the active participation of Africans as labourers in the colonial economy. In practice, colonial authorities spent only the bare minimum on public health that was necessary to reproduce the labour power of Africans. Here, it bears reiterating that health promotion and protection initiatives were almost always designed to exclusively benefit Europeans.

This raises questions of equity, justice and fairness. Of course, it seems to be a contradiction in terms to expect 'equity, fairness and justice' from colonialism. Yet, it is worth noting that colonial authorities frequently invoked such ideological goals to justify colonialism. These goals include, 'socio-political emancipation,' 'enlightenment,' and 'civilization'—all concepts that incorporate some aspect of equity, justice and fairness. As John Rawls argued in his authoritative work on the justice question, no meaningful conceptualization of justice allows that anyone be denied freedom to ensure attainment of the greater good for others. Therefore, the colonial practice of employing scarce resources to address exclusively the health needs of Europeans was indefensible on this score.

Colonialism, like imperialism before it, drew much of its inspiration from the belief that the White race was culturally and racially superior to 'racial others.' Policies that prioritized the health or other needs of Europeans over those of others were informed by this belief or ideology. Here, I hasten to underscore the fact that race is not a biological concept. Rather, it is an ideology, whose definition is conditioned by circumstances. For a long time, especially during the heydays of colonialism in Africa, it served as a force behind power relations between the conquerors and the conquered. Racism justifies the disparaging and unjust treatment of the conquered. The basis for this is the unsubstantiated belief that the conquerors are entitled to preferential and privileged treatment because of their alleged superiority.

The same ideology also constitutes the foundation of the narrow definition of the concept of public interest, which was essentially tantamount to the special interests of the colonial powers. It is safe to state that all decisions in colonial Africa were designed to serve some special interest of colonial master nations. Meyerson and Banfield (1955) expressed this more eloquently. A decision qualifies as serving special interests if it seeks to advance the interests of some part of a given public at the expense of the interests of the larger segment of that public. Most colonial public health policies were designed to address the health needs of the few Europeans resident in the colonial territories. In fact, all policies by the colonial state in Africa were designed to serve no more than a special interest of some sort.

If, as Thomas Hobbes once argued, the state constitutes a contract between the individual and government, one cannot but wonder whether it is accurate to talk of a state in colonial Africa. The thought of a state in this context seems absurd given that there was never any contract between Africans and the colonial states that European colonial powers imposed on them in the nineteenth century. Naomi Chazan and her colleagues (1992) have presented one of the most authoritative statements on the state in colonial Africa. Their description of the administrative structure of the colonial bureaucratic machinery is particularly informative.

This machinery was hierarchically ordered in the classic Weberian sense. Thus, within any given colony, the administrative and other colonial government functions were concentrated in the hands of the colonial civil service located in the administrative capital city of that colony. Also worthy of note is the fact that the machinery was typically organized along functional lines. Thus, a colonial administrative system would typically comprise a government unit in charge of health, public security and the enforcement of law and order, public works, and revenue collection. The responsibility for public health was often divided mainly between the units in charge of health and public works. This latter was typically placed in charge of sanitation infrastructure development and maintenance. In some cases, whole departments were created and placed specifically in charge of sanitation. One case in point is that of colonial Lagos, where a Sanitary Department—complete with a Sanitary Engineer and an Inspector of Nuisance—was established in 1888 (Bigon, 2005).

Within the colonial politico-administrative framework, the role for policy formulation was often relegated to authorities in the metropole or colonial master nation. This was more the rule than the exception in colonies under French control. The proclivity for centralizing administrative structures has always been a defining feature of the French. Alexis de Tocqueville, in *Democracy in America*, had drawn attention to this tendency as far back as 1835. Then, de Tocqueville had remarked that France under Louis XIV possessed the most centralized politico-administrative structure of all Western polities (de Tocqueville, 1835: 41-44). When the French began their colonial venture in Africa in the late-1800s, they were quick to insist on centralized administrative structures as the ideal mechanisms for attaining their colonial development goals. On their part, the British tended to institute a more or less decentralized politico-administrative structure. This structure dictated that local chiefs and headmen play a critical role in the day-to-day affairs of colonial governance. This system is what came to be widely known as 'indirect rule' in contrast to the 'direct rule' strategy of the French and to some extent, the Portuguese. Indirect rule, was most efficient in locales with a pre-colonial history of centralized power structures, and/or established kingdoms or chiefdoms. In the acephalous or stateless polities, which had a history of decentralized authority, the British found it necessary to 'invent' centralized authorities. These came to be known as 'warrant chiefs' as in the case in colonial southeastern Nigeria.

The type of organizational structure determined to a large extent the type of ideology that shaped public health policies in the colonies. For instance, in the territories under direct rule, these policies drew most of their inspiration from the relevant dominant ideologies in the metropole. In contrast, public health policies in 'indirectly ruled' territories were, to a considerable extent, influenced by 'indigenous elitism.' Such policies bore the ideological traces of African elites. Two major types of elites existed in Africa during the initial phase of the colonial era. The first, I refer to as the indigenous elites, while the second I label, the invented elites. The indigenous elite included local kings, chiefs, and priests, who were in charge of social, political and religious affairs during the pre-colonial era. The invented elites included those that gravitated to prominence as a result of allying with colonial authorities, adopting the 'modern' ways of life, and especially obtaining formal education. In French colonies the invented elites were also known as '*les evolués*.' The invented elites played a prominent role in Westernizing health and sanitation principles and practices in Africa during the colonial era and beyond. Witness for instance, the role of the minority missionary-educated elite known as the Saro's in colonial Lagos (Bigon, 2005). Most of the Saro's were immigrants from Sierra Leone. This invented elite group was instrumental in supplanting indigenous sanitation practices in colonial Lagos with British varieties. Here, as Bigon (2005) observed, the invented elite displayed less patience than British colonial authorities with the slow pace at which efforts to Europeanize colonial Lagos from a public health and sanitation perspective were proceeding in the 1880s (Bigon, 2005).

The task of policy implementation in the colonies involved unscrupulous tactics. These tactics entailed mainly manipulation, coercion, and outright brutality by military forces. Military force was frequently used to ensure compliance with specific dictates and to brutally deal with expressions of dissatisfaction with colonial government policy. From this vantage point, the colonial state can be considered, for all practical purposes, a military administrative unit. More noteworthy is the fact that it contained all elements of an authoritarian state. In this light, the colonial state was never involved in any consultation as a prelude to, or part of the policy or decision making process. The need to appreciate these aspects of the colonial state is accentuated by the fact that it constituted the nucleus around which the post-colonial state was constructed. The administrative structure of this state is what indigenous authorities inherited on the eve of independence throughout Africa. The inherited institutions were impoverished, subversive of the public interest and externally controlled. The indigenous leadership inherited not only the colonial administrative structures, but also, colonial government laws and policies. Consequently, the post-colonial era has been characterized more by continuity than change. This has had far-reaching implications for policymaking in many sectors, and particularly public health. This is evident in the various ideologies that have shaped public health elements of urban planning in Africa during the colonial era and subsequent to the demise of colonialism.

Yet, no ideology was as influential as the race ideology in shaping the nature of health elements of urban planning in colonial Africa. The formal onset of the colonial era in Africa is 1884/85. This is when European colonial powers decided, at a conference that was held in Berlin, to divide the continent amongst themselves. The prevailing ideology of the colonial era in Africa was one of White racial superiority; and the popular view was that Africans were not only racially inferior but were sub-human and dispensable. This view constituted the basis for policies that sought to improve health conditions in exclusive European enclaves while ignoring the health problems of African settlements. The massive efforts that were summoned to tackle malaria in European tropical colonies such as Sierra Leone exemplify this tendency.

It is also worth noting for the purpose of this discussion that within the framework of the racist thinking of the colonial era, Africans were perceived as vectors of disease. This view held sway and became the basis of many colonial spatial development policies. Despite evidence challenging its therapeutic value, no efforts were ever made to reverse or discontinue racial residential segregation policies in tropical Africa. In fact, many authoritative studies had uncovered evidence debunking the baseless theories that incriminated Africans as the vectors of lethal disease-causing agents. For instance, in 1881, Carlos Finlay had discovered that mosquitoes—and not Africans—were the vector for yellow fever. This was long before racial residential segregation became an official colonial 'health policy.' Alfonse Lavernan as well as other scientists in France, Italy, England, and the United States also uncovered information that exonerated Africans as the vectors of malaria. The fact that proponents of racial residential segregation as a health promotion/protection strategy were not persuaded by this preponderance of evidence is telling. It suggests that the racist ideology of the time and not science constituted the basis for public health policy making. Here, the manner in which the findings of Dr. Ronald Ross and his associates at the Liverpool School of Tropical Medicine were employed constitutes a glaring testament (see Frenkel and Western, 1988; Njoh, 2008). According to the findings, the *Anopheles* mosquito carried *Plasmodia*, the malaria parasite, and then passes it through one stage of development within the mosquito, and another within the human host. This revelation was used by Joseph Chamberlain, the British Colonial Secretary to rationalize his edict to racially segregate all British colonies in Tropical Africa (Frenkel and Western 1988).

### The state, ideology, health and planning in contemporary Africa

Most analyses of the state have focalized on advanced nations. Thus, despite its pre-eminence, the state in Africa is seldom the object of analysis by social scientists and others interested in African development. Chazan and her colleagues (1992) have expressed similar sentiments. Elsewhere, I have also observed that "the African state ... continues to be virtually ignored in discussions of the African political economy" (Njoh, 2003: 6). Resulting from this virtual neglect has been a lack of adequate appreciation for the nature, form, and role of the state in Africa. Yet, it is well established that the colonial state constitutes the basis of the post-colonial state in Africa (Chazan et al., 1992). Like the colonial state, the postcolonial state tends to operate without legitimacy. Consequently, it has, like its predecessor, the colonial state, frequently resorted to the use of force. Also, it has had to operate on a paltry budget. Moreover, it has been manipulated by external forces, residing mainly in the erstwhile colonial master nations. Thus, as we shall see, some of the policies that African governments have enacted to address public health problems have been dictated not by internal conditions but by external forces.

Some aspects of the theories discussed above in relation to the state in colonial Africa are also applicable to the state in contemporary African society. For example, borrowing from Marxist theoretical formulations, it can be argued that the state in Africa is by no means a fair-minded arbiter of change. Rather, it has its own interests that it constantly seeks to protect. It does this by means of its many actions and inactions in society. The modern African state is said to possess a number of major features, with the most prominent being the following (Njoh, 2003: 16; Mazrui, 1986): centralization of authority, centralized power, a fiscal system of some sort, and a supervised judiciary system. Centralization of authority, a colonial legacy, served to guarantee the level of security that the indigenous leadership needed to govern disparate ethnic groups forced to co-exist in polities that were hastily carved out by European colonial powers. In this regard, Donald Gordon (2001: 68) remarked,"from the outset, the leadership of most new states [in Africa] felt—and indeed were—politically insecure ... most of the new governments had only a thin base of support after unravelling of the anticolonial alliances left those in power with limited backing" (often of only their own ethnic groups and regions).

Centralization was also rationalized by those who inherited the colonial states in Africa as a means of ensuring national unity and economic development. Furthermore, the propensity for centralization during the immediate post-colonial era is a function of the fact that the indigenous leadership continued to rely on administrative systems and consultants from the West. Finally, it is important to note that centralization of authority is a critical aspect of the classic Weberian or bureaucratic model. This feature serves an important function, namely ensuring supervision and coordination through a carefully defined hierarchy of superiors.

Until the IMF/World Bank-initiated Structural Adjustment Programmes of the 1980s/1990s, the state in Africa was virtually responsible for the delivery of all social services. Thus, the indigenous leaders were expected, among other things, to address the socio-economic needs of their growing populations. was African leaders were also expected to initiate and institute national development programmes. To appreciate this as a tall order, one needs to simply acknowledge the fact that the colonial governance structures that indigenous authorities inherited were designed to achieve relatively less complicated tasks. These tasks included the collection of taxes, the maintenance of law and order, and the provisioning of basic services.

The many weaknesses of colonial governance structures became evident soon after the demise of the colonial era. These weaknesses were amplified as the colonial state apparatus was required to promote national development. The deficiency of this apparatus was most pronounced in sectors with tasks and responsibilities that were unknown during the colonial era. The health sector constitutes a good example in this regard. Here, the definition of the word 'public' in public health was no longer limited to a very small segment of the population, namely the Europeans. Rather, the term had to be broadened to encompass everyone in the towns, cities and villages of the newly-independent countries. The indigenous leadership therefore faced a more complicated problem. This problem had to do with the acute shortage of skilled personnel. Writing in the 1960s, when almost all African countries secured political independence, Albert Waterston (1965) noted that efforts to "Africanize the bureaucracy" were thwarted by the problem of finding enough qualified Africans. More than two decades later, many analysts were still echoing Waterston's observation by noting the dire shortage of skills in Africa (see e.g., Njoh, 1990).

The severe shortage of skilled workers did not translate into bureaucracies with few employees. In fact, the contrary was true. A unique feature of the post-colonial state in Africa is the fact that it has always been dominated and controlled by a very small segment of society. During the colonial era, this small segment was comprised of the few colonial authorities and other Europeans based in the colonial territories. Today, this segment consists of a handful of privileged indigenous elements, often referred to as the ruling class. This class wields and employs enormous power to advance its own self-defined organizational, political and economic interests (Njoh, 1999). For this reason, some analysts view the state in Africa as an effective tool for resource accumulation that has always been employed by a largely decadent, unproductive and corrupt dominant class to advance its own self-interests (see e.g., Ihonvbere, 1994). Thus, contrary to the situation in advanced capitalist societies, where the state may be employed for purposes of legitimization, the state in Africa is employed for the purpose of accumulation and ultimately self-aggrandizement. More worthy of note is the fact that, on the one hand, the ruling class is not hesitant to "employ the structures, institutions and instruments of the state to repress, exploit, suppress, and marginalize the masses" (Njoh, 1999: 112). On the other hand, the masses perceive "the state as nothing other than an exploitative, coercive and alien entity that must be treated with suspicion at best and fear and contempt at worst" (p.112).

Although characterizing the state as 'exploitative' and 'coercive' may be a little harsh, it is arguable that its actions in any given policy field are designed to first and foremost satisfy one or another of its myriad interests. This position constitutes the thrust of the argument presented in this book. Essentially, it is argued that the constellation of actions that governments throughout Africa have taken with the avowed aim of improving public health in the built environment are designed to ultimately address the state's interests. While these interests may be vast, only those with an ideological bent are of concern here. A quick examination of some public health elements of urban planning on the continent is necessary to illuminate this point.

The ideology in vogue in Africa during the twilight of the European colonial era, and for about two decades following independence, in most of the countries was modernization. Modernization theory emerged after World War II and served as the dominant scholarly and professional response to the development problematic in Africa and other developing regions. The major tenets of modernization theory revolved around four main assumptions (Latham, 2000; Udogu, Online; Harrison, 1988; Mclelland, 1961; Inkeles and Smith, 1974; Rostow, 1961). These include the fact that: 1) 'traditional' (i.e. non-Western societies including all erstwhile colonies) and 'modern' (i.e. Western societies, particularly the former colonial master nations) societies are distinct; 2) economic, political, and social changes are inextricably intertwined; 4) development tends to proceed toward the modern state along a common, linear path; and 4) progress in traditional societies can be achieved if and only if they maintain contact with modern societies. Contact with modern societies was necessary but not sufficient for traditional societies to become modern. Rather, to become modern, traditional societies needed to mimic the socio-economic, political and technological strategies that have been adopted by their modern counterparts.

The thrust of modernization theory is that societies can be arranged to form a pyramid in which the apex is occupied by the erstwhile colonial master nations of Europe and other industrialized countries, particularly the United States. Most members of the intellectual and international development policy communities at the time believed that the lessons of the erstwhile colonial powers' past demonstrate without equivocation the route to genuine modernity. Accordingly, they recommended that the newly independent countries of Africa (as well as other so-called 'traditional,' 'stagnant,' or 'underdeveloped' societies) strive to emulate the achievements of the former colonial powers.

When it came to addressing the health consequences of the rapid population growth that was occurring throughout Africa at the time, authorities were advised to simply duplicate the efforts of Europeans. Earlier on in the mid-nineteenth century, Europeans had had occasion to deal with the health challenges of the industrial revolution. For instance, in England, the work of social reformers such as Edwin Chadwick and Friedrich Engels had accentuated the need for policymakers to be attentive to the health consequences of population growth and concomitant changes especially in urban areas. Chadwick's 1842 'Report on the Sanitary Conditions of the Labouring Population of Great Britain' (Chadwick, 1842) and Engels's 1844 work, 'Conditions of the Working Classes in 1844' (Engels, 1844) linked living conditions and amenities to disease. These and other efforts had led to the enactment of Britain's maiden Public Health Act in 1848. This Act or elements thereof were adopted throughout Western Europe. Most of the efforts in this regard were directed at housing and environmental design.

Since the 1990s, the ideology that has influenced health elements of urban planning in Africa has been globalism or globalization. Although globalism and globalization are sometimes used interchangeably, the two concepts are fundamentally distinct (Locke, 2003). On the one hand globalization is an inevitable phenomenon, which in recent times has manifested itself in the growth of communication, trade, and South-North migration. On the other hand, "globalism is an ideology, a set of opinions about how things ought to be" (Locke, para. 1). Globalists attribute no role to the state. Rather, they see the world functioning as one seamless unit governed by the same rules under the auspices of trans-national non-governmental entities such as the World Trade Organization (WTO), the International Bank for Reconstruction and Development (the World Bank), and the World Health Organization (WHO). Threads of globalism manifest themselves in health elements of urban planning through programmes of these and other international development organizations. Examples of such programmes include the 'Healthy Cities' and cognate initiatives such as 'Safe Cities,' both of which fall under the auspices of the UN. These and similar programmes constitute part of efforts on the part of Western international development agencies. Their aim is to accomplish the ideological mission of universalizing Eurocentric notions of health in the built environment.

### Ideology, public health and the sustainability question

The sustainability of public health in general and hygiene and sanitation systems in particular, is best illustrated by the schemes that indigenous elites promoted during the pre-colonial era. As an ideological basis for formulating hygiene and sanitation policies, indigenous elitism contributed the least towards hampering or complicating Africa's development efforts. What the indigenous elites set out to accomplish in hygiene and sanitation, and the means they employed were contextually relevant. After all, indigenous elites were intimately familiar with the realities of the environment in which they functioned. Also, they were products of that environment. To be sure, the policies enacted by indigenous elites were not without blemish. Some of these policies had obvious limitations or negative implications. For instance, refuse disposal through burning could contribute to ailments such as respiratory tract infections. Also, the attribution of all diseases to acts of God was rather too simplistic. Beliefs such as these possessed the potential to thwart efforts to locate the actual causes of public health problems.

Yet, it is necessary to note that traditional strategies incorporated elements of African traditions. Thus, they were more contextually relevant than the imported alternatives. The incorporation of aspects of African culture such as taboos, norms and beliefs relating to environmental pollution, hygiene and sanitation in the public health policies they crafted is but only one testament to this. Citizen participation was mandated for the implementation of most hygiene and sanitation policies of the pre-colonial era. Such a requirement was rooted in the ruling elites' knowledge of the indigenous African ethos of communalism. The following argument is therefore logical in this light. The received hygiene and sanitation policies promulgated by indigenous elites were defined by African tradition, culture, and beliefs. Consequently, they were more contextual and more sustainable than those enacted by colonial and post-colonial authorities. The role of context and prevailing conditions is critical here. For instance, while good housing can potentially enhance public health, it is incapable of succeeding on this score if prevailing economic, social and cultural conditions are ignored or discounted. Good housing entails a lot more than just four walls and a roof. It also entails a lot more than the use of so-called modern building materials. It encompasses issues relating to broader aspects of the environment such as its ability to guarantee the safety, security and emotional serenity of its inhabitants.

The more contextual hygiene and sanitation strategies of indigenous Africans became a casualty of the ideology of modernization. In other words, this ideology and the concomitant tendency on the part of Europeans to downplay the accomplishments of Africans conspired to prevent colonial authorities from taking advantage of the medical expertise of Africans at the time. Although more than half a century has elapsed since these schemes were implemented, they continue to hamper development efforts on the continent. The spatially-based health policies that were founded on the modernization ideology have had equally far-reaching negative implications for contemporary development efforts throughout the continent. For instance, the compartmentalization of land use activities, or zoning, as a means of promoting public health has served to elongate the distance between activity points. This has significantly increased the cost of transportation. Similarly, the implementation of policies to eradicate so-called slums has resulted in increasing the cost of housing. This is because destroying the so-called slums effectively results in diminishing the stock of residential units.

The tendency to treat so-called slums and informal settlements with disdain is itself a function of two inextricably intertwined ideologies, namely modernism and Euro-centricity. The former equates 'old' with 'obsolescence.' The latter considers non-Western practices, concepts and technology as 'primitive,' 'dysfunctional' and 'antithetical to development.' Consider the following. In a recent and otherwise rich survey of slums in global perspectives, Mike Davis characterizes slums as overcrowded, poor, unhygienic, and insalubrious human settlements whose inhabitants are mainly involved in 'racket' or 'criminal trade' (Davis, 2006: 12).

It is hard to miss the searing condemnation of so-called slums imbibed in the foregoing characterization. Such condemnation and concomitant policies that have sought to eradicate slums are by no means new. What is of recent vintage are the gargantuan size and rapid rate of growth of slum settlements in developing countries. As Davis (2006: 13) notes, 78 percent (78.2%) of the urban population of the least developed countries and a third of the global urban population live in slums. In some African countries such as Ethiopia and Chad, almost all of the urban population live in slums (Ibid).

The modernization ideology is also responsible for causing a number of other socio-economic problems in Africa. For instance, proponents of modernization advocate the exclusive use of Euro-centric building materials as a public health measure. Possible consequences of this include capital flight and heavy losses in foreign exchange as Africans are compelled to import building materials. Another result of the policies is that they have led to gender-based income disparities. This is because the use of Euro-centric building materials and techniques is biased in favour of men, who are the ones involved in the so-called modern building trades (masonry, electricity, plumbing, tile hanging, etc). Here, it is necessary to note that this bias is a product of 'modernization.' In contrast to what obtained in Europe especially in Victorian England, pre-colonial African women were very active in all sectors including construction (Njoh, 2006).

Globalism as an ideological basis for spatially based public health policies has real and potential negative implications for development efforts in Africa. Consider, for instance, the clarion call by proponents of the concept of 'healthy cities' to develop special areas and facilities, such as recreational parks, jogging/ cycling trails, and sporting arenas for physical exercise. While such a call is logical in industrialized societies, they are illogical and unrealistic in African countries for many reasons. First, while industrialized countries possess the financial resources necessary for implementing such projects, African countries do not. Second, in contrast to the situation in Africa, the nature of daily activities in industrialized societies, particularly the excessive reliance on motorized means of transportation, renders passive exercise difficult. Finally, most areas are built-up thereby raising the premium on parks and green spaces as critical environmental amenities in industrialized countries (Frumkin, 2005). However, this is not the case in Africa where undeveloped land remains plentiful in many parts.

A more far-reaching implication of healthy cities programmes in Africa is their reliance on foreign aid. The record of foreign aid in Africa leaves much to be desired. African countries have very little to show despite having been beneficiaries of foreign aid since the end of World War II. Instead, as critics (e.g., Bauer, 1984) contend, it is obvious that foreign aid has created extensive opportunities for rent seeking for African leaders. Additionally, foreign aid has led to the politicization of poverty. Politicians are wont to consolidate power by using foreign aid funds as a tool for rewarding allies and punishing enemies. In fact, some critics of foreign aid have gone so far as to suggest as follows. Foreign aid is responsible for demoting Africa from a food exporter to a continent in which many countries currently lack the ability to feed their population (e.g., Sowell, 1983; Bauer, 1984; Ayittey, 1988). The foregoing suggests three possible real and/or potential problems of foreign aid in the healthy cities programme. First, there is the likelihood of politicians using foreign aid resources to support healthy cities projects only in towns and urban centres considered allies. Conversely, they would withhold funds from regions they consider 'enemies', of the ruling regime. Second, there is also the possibility of foreign aid serving as a disincentive to self-reliant initiatives. For instance, citizens may insist on being paid for their participation in projects funded by foreign. Such citizens were likely to have considered their participation as a civic duty otherwise. Finally, despite claims to the contrary, the foreign aid donors invariably influence the agenda of healthy cities authorities in the aid recipient countries. Thus, the means and strategies employed to implement healthy cities projects are important. Their outcomes reflect and embody the norms, ideals, values and predilections of the Western aid benefactor as opposed to those of Africans.

Ideologically-based policies are neither novel nor unique to Africa. Most policies in the developed world have ideological roots. In fact, capitalism, upon which many policies in the West are based, is itself an ideology. Yet, the fact that the policies repose on an ideological foundation has not resulted in their failure. It is therefore necessary to re-examine any theory that incriminates ideology as a menace to development. In the case of Africa, I submit that it is not ideology per se, but its source (endogenous versus exogenous), that is more likely to hamper development. In other words, a development policy is more likely to fail when it is based on an imported ideology than when it is rooted in ideology of the indigenous variety. Ideally, however, meaningful development policy must be driven by genuine science and a desire to promote development rather than by ideology.

## Conclusion

We would be remiss if we ended this chapter without emphasizing the need to reinvigorate the link between spatial structures and public health. It is also necessary to underscore the importance of reintegrating public health into urban planning policies in Africa. However, it is necessary to stress that the decision to adopt any health promotion or hygiene and sanitation strategy must repose more on sound science tempered with a good dose of pragmatism and less on ideology. In this latter case, indigenous ideology must be weighted more heavily than ideology of the imported variety. This suggests that planners in Africa would do well to either make an effort to 'Africanize' received hygiene and sanitation elements of planning policies. In other words such policies should be endowed with attributes of African culture. Alternatively, only those policies that already possess such attributes should be adopted. Promoting farming, a well-established African tradition, as a public health element of urban planning exemplifies strategies of the latter genre. Urban agriculture, an early casualty of so-called modern urban development strategies, was formally recognized for its contribution to urban public health and welfare during the UN International Conference on Human Settlements in Istanbul in 1996. It is said to possess several health benefits, including but not limited to the following (Bellows, Brown and Smit, Online):

- Growing food correlates strongly with food consumption, which is important for good health;
- The active work necessary for meaningful urban agriculture serves as an important recreational activity for urban dwellers;
- Urban agriculture contributes to the creation of green areas, which are essential for enhancing urban public health.

Pragmatism dictates that efforts be made to ensure that public health elements of urban policies are sensitive to their context. Perhaps more importantly, policymakers must be alert to the inescapable forces of globalization, which tend to generate new challenges of their own. For instance, the forces of globalization threaten to aggravate urban health and safety problems (Suresh, 2003). Prominent in this regard are obvious problems such as those associated with environmental pollution and natural resource degradation. In addition those rooted in emerging environmental forces such as global warming and ozone depletion. Success in addressing the future problems of cities will depend largely on the extent to which deliberate and systematic efforts and resources are marshalled to accomplish the following objectives (cf., Suresh, 2003; Davis, 2006):

- Improved access to potable water, sanitation and drainage facilities;
- Improved systems for solid waste disposal;
- Reduced levels of pollution and clean air; and
- Significantly reduced levels of poverty.

The last objective, reducing levels of poverty, is particularly important for one particular reason—the fact that poverty is at the root of most problems, including poor sanitation services, environmental degradation and inadequate health facilities. The poverty status of slum dwellers means that they do not constitute a viable source of municipal revenue. Consequently, municipal authorities are unable to provide or maintain sanitation services and infrastructure in slums. Thus, to eradicate poverty is to promote public health. However, while the elimination of poverty is necessary, it is not sufficient as a strategy for addressing the health problems of African urban areas now and in the future. Authorities would do well to blend together foreign and indigenous human settlement development strategies, policies and practices that are economically and socio-culturally sustainable while capable of guaranteeing the health, safety and security of their inhabitants.

# Chapter 3

# Town Planning, Public Health and the Colonial Project

## Introduction

As stated in Chapter 1, the professions of town planning and public health emerged in response to a common problem—the health consequences of the industrial revolution. Efforts in both professions to wrestle with cholera and other epidemics in Europe from 1830 to 1880 is further testament to their shared goals. During this period, planning focused intensely on functionality and hierarchical ordering of land use through zoning. The overriding goal here, at least in theory, was to promote public health by regulating the type of contact occurring between people and land use activities. When the colonial era began in Africa, European town planners wasted no time in transplanting to the continent schemes that had been developed to address the health consequences of the industrial revolution and the concomitant expansion of urban populations in Europe. There is hardly any paucity of knowledge on the process by which the transfer of planning knowledge from Europe to Africa occurred (see e.g., Njoh, 2002; Chokor, 1993; Simon, 1992; King, 1990; 1976; Kanyeihamba, 1980; Abu-Lughod, 1965). Also, there is a growing body of literature on the implications for development of employing European town planning schemes in Africa (see e.g., Njoh, 2003; 1999; King, 1990). However, with a few exceptions (e.g., Frenkel and Western, 1988; Curtin, 1985), little has been done to explore the ulterior motives of the many schemes that were implemented throughout Africa under the pretext of promoting public health. Far less has been done to explore the ideological foundations of these schemes and their implications for development efforts in post-colonial Africa. Consequently, there is a vast gap in our knowledge of how public health served as a pretext for attaining other important objectives of the colonial project in Africa. This chapter is intended as a modest contribution to efforts dedicated to bridging this gap. Knowledge of colonial public health initiatives in Africa is crucial not only for historical purposes. Rather, such knowledge is invaluable because the schemes constitute the nucleus around which contemporary public health policy and infrastructure on the continent have been developed.

## Public health as an element of colonial town planning

Quite early during the colonial era, authorities decided in favour of controlling all aspects of urban life in their tropical African colonies. Accordingly, the powers of the police, sanitation inspectors, and mayors were all reinforced. This reinforcement constituted an expansion of the state apparatus or the exercise of a form of power akin to what Foucault (1982) has characterized as 'pastoral power.' Pastoral power in the Foucaultian sense focuses on salvation, particularly with respect to reforming people's health or habits and the use of 'individualizing techniques' (Yeoh, 2003). In noting similar dynamics within the colonial urban environment of Singapore, Brenda Yeoh contended that the British colonial authorities had created and charged several institutions with the task of urban governance. Yeoh further argued that "although each institution had its own 'field operation,' they shared the use of common disciplinary forms to mould the colonized body and the space it inhabited so as to facilitate social order and economic advancement, the twin imperatives which supplied the rationale for action and which came to dominate colonial policy" (Yeoh, 2003: 11).

Health concerns constituted the official rationale for most Town Planning schemes that were implemented in colonial Africa. Some of the most prominent of the public health schemes that were executed during the colonial era in Africa have been exhaustively discussed by Curtin (1985). The schemes can be appreciated under the following three broad categories according to their avowed purposes, namely malaria combating strategies; plague control and combating; and general hygiene and public health promotion (see Table 3.1).

## Table 3.1 Major health components of urban planning, colonial Africa

| Item | Avowed Aim of Scheme | Specific Planning Activity |
|------|----------------------|----------------------------|
| A. | Malaria Combating | Racial spatial segregation;<br>Ample ventilation of housing units;<br>Elimination of mosquito breeding places (e.g., standing water and overgrown vegetation);<br>Location of European settlements on high altitudes;<br>Nocturnal racial segregation. |
| B. | Plague Combating | Quarantining or isolation of infected populations;<br>Relocation of infected members of the indigenous populations to locales far-removed from European settlements;[1]<br>Burning down African villages or African sections of urban centers suspected of being infected.[2] |
| C. | General hygiene and public health promotion | Destruction of so-called squalid and dilapidated buildings;<br>Enforcement of building codes and ordinances;<br>Regulation of the timing and location of objects in the built environment under the rubric of zoning;<br>Regulation of noise levels under the auspices of noise pollution and nuisance ordinances and laws;<br>Prohibition of the development of African traditional building structures (e.g. thatch/earth units) from urban areas. |

*Notes*: [1] For example from September to October 1914, 2,900 Africans were expelled from Dakar. Similarly, in Douala, the Germans initiated a mass relocation scheme to move all natives from the area around the sea to hinterland areas; there is also the case of such an attempt to relocate natives en masse from Mombassa and Nairobi, respectively to hinterland areas (see Curtin, 1985, p. 611). [2] One case in point is that of Dakar, 1914 (see Curtin, 1985, p. 608).

*Malaria combating schemes*

From the early- to mid-nineteenth century, it was widely believed that particular locations, soils, temperature and rainfall were all determinants of health conditions. In other words, the health status of a place was considered a function of its location (on the hill or in a valley); the characteristic of the soil at the place (loose versus hard soil, dry versus wet soil); the temperature of the place (hot or cold); and the extent or degree of rainfall at the place (heavy or light). This belief is one of a number of rationales that were advanced in defense of the selection of higher ground, especially hilltops, as the location of choice for European residential and colonial administrative facilities. In fact, stipulations to the effect that housing for military personnel and Europeans in, especially colonial Africa, India, and the West Indies be located on higher ground and/or placed on stilts and elevated to ten to fifteen feet above ground were rooted in this belief (Curtin, 1985). On the one hand, higher altitudes, it was believed for centuries, translated to cooler weather, which was in turn associated with good health. On the other hand, lower elevation was associated with warm or hot weather, which in turn translated into putrefaction and hence, disease.

This belief, it turned out, was in error. However, it was certainly not the only erroneous assumption at the foundation of most public health policies in colonial Africa. Another erroneous decision with implications for spatial organization in general and town planning laws in particular in Africa had to do with malaria. To be sure, malaria has always been a lethal tropical disease. The medical wisdom of the time held that the source of malaria was the soil. Writing in 1834, F. H. Rankin, had characterized malaria as a disease "caused by emanations from the soil, which crept 'assasin-like close to the earth'" (quoted in Curtin, 1985: 594). It was also erroneously believed that African adults possessed some type of immunity against malaria. This conclusion was derived from a number of studies revealing that blood samples from African adults rarely contained actual plasmodia. On the contrary, the blood of children manifesting clinical symptoms contained this parasite. Therefore, the malaria experts of the time concluded, African children, and not adults, were the primary source of malarial infection. However, this and identical characterizations of the source of malaria were later to be debunked by works identifying the anopheles mosquito as the vector of this lethal disease.

British town planning in colonial Africa drew a lot of its inspiration from the British colonial experience in India. Particularly noteworthy for the purpose of the present discussion are the sanitation reform measures that were instituted in India and later transplanted to colonial Africa. The best known of these measures are those that were adopted in 1863 to address health problems created by the Sepoy Mutiny of 1857 and the Crimean War (Curtin, 1985). One aspect of these reforms that was later transplanted to colonial Africa is the cantonment system which was established in the 1870s and 1880s (Ibid, 1985: 595). Using health concerns as a pretext, colonial authorities moved to construct permanent military camps in locations far removed from the native areas. Such locations, these authorities argued, were necessary to isolate British military personnel from the "noxious ordours of native habitation" (Ibid: 595). The same argument was advanced to rationalize the construction of military barracks in British colonial Africa. Here, the development of residential units for colonial officials and other Europeans in the colonies followed the same pattern. Apart from their isolated locations, these units possessed another noteworthy feature that distinguished them from native housing, namely excessive ventilation. Ventilation and air quality were accorded a priority place on the health policy agenda of colonial authorities. This is because the authorities believed that "generalized contagion might build up to dangerous levels without a constant change of air" (Curtin, 1985: 597, citing Rosenberg, 1977). These ideas however, began to rapidly change with advancements in germ sciences. One discovery, credited to Louis Pasteur and Robert Koch, in this connection revealed that some diseases are caused by bacteria that invade and live on an organism as parasites.

New germ theories such as the foregoing prepared the stage for a lot of noteworthy works. These works significantly influenced health and spatial policies in tropical Africa. Perhaps the most prominent development in this regard is Carlos Finlay's discovery in 1881 that mosquitoes were the vector for yellow fever. In this regard, the mosquitoes carried the yellow fever parasite from person to person. Philip Curtin (1985: 597) draws attention to a number of other major works that served to bolster Finlay's theory. Worth noting in this regard were the discovery by Alfonse Lavernan of malaria parasites in the blood of malaria patients. Further evidence corroborating this theory came from France, Italy, England and the United States. In England, particularly at the Liverpool School of Tropical Medicine, Ronald Ross and his colleagues had concluded that the *Anopheles* mosquito carried the *Plasmodia*, the malaria parasite, which passed through one stage of development within the mosquito and another within the human host.

In 1899, Ross and a number of his colleagues were dispatched to Sierra Leone, a bastion for malaria. Their mission was to conduct studies ascertaining that the Anopheles mosquito was indeed the vector for malaria in Africa. The researchers conducted two malaria control experiments in Sierra Leone, one in 1899 and another in 1900 (Frenkel and Western, 1988). In addition to establishing with certainty the link between the Anopheles mosquito and malaria, the researchers made one additional discovery. They determined that the Anopheles mosquito did most of its biting and infection at night and not during the day. Therefore, as a public health strategy, only nocturnal segregation of the European from the indigenous population was necessary. In practice, the scientists argued, it was possible for Europeans and members of the indigenous population to work together as long as they were spatially separated at night. Thus, Europeans could work and visit indigenous areas of the town during day. However, they must return to their homes in the European districts at night. Similarly, servants, gardeners and others could work in the European districts at night and return to the indigenous settlements at night. These recommendations appear fastidious at best. In this regard, colonial authorities conveniently failed to acknowledge the fact that some workers, such as night watchmen had to spend the night in the European districts. Soon after Ross and his colleagues reported their findings and recommendations, Joseph Chamberlain, the Colonial Secretary at the time pronounced racial residential segregation as official policy in all of Britain's tropical African colonies.

Among his many recommendations, Ross had opined that the best way to deal with the malaria problem in Africa was to adopt the cantonment policy. He noted that this system had been successfully used in British colonial India.

Accordingly, he recommended that housing for Europeans be located at least two kilometers from indigenous settlements. This was based on two main, seemingly contradictory, assumptions. First, it was believed, albeit erroneously, that the African Anopheles mosquito preferred the blood of Africans as opposed to that of Europeans. Hence, the mosquito would have a propensity for flying within African settlements regardless of the distance they are capable of traversing. Second, scientific knowledge of the time suggested that, factoring in the possibility of being assisted by wind, the Anopheles mosquito could not traverse a distance in excess of two kilometers.

As a public health promotion strategy, it was not enough, colonial authorities believed, to simply isolate European residential units from indigenous settlements. Medical scientists such as Robert Koch, who had had extensive experience in Asia and had conducted a number of studies on malaria and blackwater fever in Africa (circa, 1897-98), recommended the prophylactic use of quinine. Others, such as S.R. Christophers and J.W.W. Stephens of the Liverpool School of Tropical Medicine considered Koch's recommendation not feasible and therefore mistaken. Colonial authorities further criticized suggestions advocating that the *Anopheles* mosquito be attacked as a means of combating malaria. Instead, they recommended that every effort be directed at singling out and protecting the Europeans.

The removal of 'susceptible Europeans' from the midst of malaria was only one of the many possible strategies rooted in recommendations such as the foregoing. Based on the erroneous belief that African children were the prime source of malarial infection, Europeans were strongly admonished against being in the vicinity of native children from zero to five years of age (Christophers and Stephens, 1980; Curtin, 1985).

The foregoing instructions were rather swiftly adopted by colonial officials on the ground in the colonies albeit to significantly different degrees. In Sierra Leone, the colonial government moved rapidly to incorporate the instructions in its spatial planning schemes, with the most conspicuous manifestations of actions in this connection being the development of the Hill Station. Work on the Hill Station in Freetown, Sierra Leone, was initiated in 1902. By1904, a considerable number of units, including the Governor's Residence, were ready for occupation. The community was developed along the lines of identical developments, also named hill stations, in British colonial India. The land for the Freetown project was confiscated from some members of the native population. Developed as an exclusively European enclave, Hill Station overlooks, and is connected to, Freetown by a narrow gauge mountain railroad (Njoh, 1999; Frenkel and Western, 1988). It is four miles removed from the main city, Freetown and only 700 feet above sea level—a far-cry from the 4 to 5000 feet altitude that was recommended to protect the health of Europeans in the colonies.

A number of peculiar features of the units in the community are worth mentioning. The units were built to face north and supported by columns several feet above ground level, while the ground beneath the buildings was covered with cement. The orientation was designed to take advantage of the air/wind pattern.

This, it was believed, permitted maximum ventilation and air circulation within the units. Raising the structure and cementing the ground beneath was believed to be a strategy for preventing 'malarial poisons' from rising from the soil and peculating into the building. This recommendation was based on archaic, anachronistic and erroneous theories that viewed the soil as the source of malaria. Hill Station was immediately surrounded by a strip of land, a quarter mile in width. The strip was cleared of all trees and tall shrubbery. Outside this strip of land was a zone, which measured one mile in width and contained tall vegetation, but in which no housing units were authorized.

Once isolated, the Europeans' residential units needed to be further protected from the mosquito and other vectors of diseases. In this regard, several measures were recommended. The first was to screen the residential units of Europeans as a means of keeping the mosquitoes out. The second was to use electric fans. Dr. Ronald Ross preferred this strategy but opposed the use of screens. He contended that screens compromised efforts to maximize ventilation. His preference for fans was on account of the fact that they served a dual purpose—keeping the body cool and driving off the mosquitoes. The third strategy was to destroy all mosquito breeding grounds in and around the Hill Station.

However, this strategy turned out to be more problematic than the colonial authorities had anticipated. The authorities were not quite conversant with the *Anopheles gambiae* and the *Anopheles funestus*, which were arguably the most dangerous of the malaria vectors in West Africa. The *A. gambiae* and the *A. funestus*, as scientific knowledge was to later reveal, could breed not only during the rainy season, in swamps or low places but also in spots as small as depressions caused by human footprints as long as they contained water for a considerable duration. This characteristic of the *A. gambiae* and the *A. funestus* made them difficult to control and distinguished them from the Caribbean Anopheles and the *Aedes Egyptae* with which the authorities were familiar. The *A. Egyptae*, the carrier of the yellow fever parasite had proven to be less problematic to control particularly because its flight range is extremely short and also because it bred in built-up areas.

The ideas of Ross, especially his staunch and unwavering opposition to the prophylactic use of quinine and fitting European houses with screens carried the day. The ideas found their way into British colonial government health policy directives. For example, as of May 1900, the Colonial Office in London began distributing pamphlets that were prepared at the Liverpool School of Tropical Medicine. The pamphlets instructed colonial officials on the ground in tropical Africa to adopt strategies to eliminate the Anopheles mosquito. As time went by, residential segregation policies were vigorously enforced as a prophylaxis against malaria.

Although colonial officials on the ground were swift in adopting these policies, the strategies and approaches they employed varied significantly in practice. In making this observation, Curtin (1985) draws attention to five specific colonies in British West Africa, namely Gambia, Sierra Leone, Gold Coast, Northern and

Southern Nigeria. In Sierra Leone, as already noted, the colonial government had decided in favour of protecting the health of members of the resident European population by segregating the races. Initially, against vehement opposition from the natives, colonial authorities had proceeded to confiscating native lands at the highest elevation. Here, they constructed a "European Only" residential area that was far-removed from the main city, Freetown. Members of the native population voiced opposition to this project. It is worth noting that, Freetown at that time contained many educated and professional Africans. In addition, it had a Black mayor. Opponents of the project were particularly critical of the horrendous sum of money that went into developing the project. They argued that the money could have been put to better use improving the city's public infrastructure. The opponents' voices fell on deaf ears as the authorities moved to implement what they contended was segregation for public health reasons. Later on, a number of other suburban projects were developed and segregated on grounds that had nothing to do with health.

In Gambia, racial residential segregation for health or any other reason for that matter was practiced on a very minimal scale. It entailed no more than the segregation of a few streets in the capital, Bathurst during World War I. Efforts to combat malaria tapped on the ideas of Koch by providing quinine free of charge to school children. This was not necessarily because the colonial authorities on the ground in Gambia were negatively predisposed to the idea of segregation. Rather, it was especially because of the scant resident European population in that colony. One account places the number of Europeans in the entire colony at one point at fewer than one hundred, with the capital city, Barthurst containing as few as twenty-two European residences (Curtin, 1985: 601). Also, members of the native population in the capital city were as economically well-off as their European counterparts. Thus, it is likely that any attempts at racial residential segregation would have met with more fierce resistance than what was encountered in Freetown. Efforts to racially segregate the upscale part of Bathurst would have entailed the prohibitively costly wholesale reconfiguration, rebuilding and redesigning of the entire area. This is because that part of town was inhabited by Europeans and wealthy Africans. For mainly these reasons, medical authorities deemed it wise abandoning any plan that would have racially segregated the city. One such plan that was called off specifically because of a lack of funds is the one to develop a segregated community for Europeans on the thirty-foot cliffs at Cape Saint Mary. This is the point at which the Gambia River enters the Atlantic Ocean. It is about 7.5 miles (about 11km) below the main city, Bathurst (Curtin, 1985: 601). In the end, authorities opted for strategies that entailed as little spatial segregation of the races as possible. One notable policy in this connection was that which called for the screening of servants' housing units but not those of their European masters. The aim here was to ensure that the ventilation of units housing Europeans was not compromised by screens. Screening the servants' quarters ensured that Europeans were not bitten by infected mosquitoes.

In Accra, Ghana, similar to the case of Bathurst, Gambia, there was a considerable number of wealthy Africans. Consequently, racial residential segregation encountered significant opposition. In fact, members of the native population were well organized and constituted a political force to reckon with. In this regard, they are on record for successfully challenging and causing the colonial government to rescind a number of potentially adverse bills, including a proposed lands bill in 1898.

Ostensibly racial residential segregation policies on health pretexts were therefore, rejected in Ghana. Instead, the colonial government in Accra moved to enact and implement alternative public health promotion town planning policies. One prominent activity in this connection was the mass demolition of so-called dilapidated buildings. Such demolition was frequently undertaken in Accra and other urban areas in the colony. Another activity in the same vain was the attempt to eradicate mosquitoes in urban areas by eliminating mosquito breeding grounds. Finally, there were a few, albeit half-hearted efforts to segregate the residential areas of government officials in Accra as well as other urban locales throughout the colony. Colonial officials in Ghana, particularly under Governor Sir Hugh Clifford, were worried that any attempt at complete segregation could have had negative consequences for race relations.

To reiterate, some colonial officials in the colonies were reluctant to implement racial residential segregation policies. The reluctance was a function of one thing. Officials in the colonies were better placed than their colleagues in the metropolitan country to appreciate the potential socio-political dangers of such policies. Nevertheless, metropolitan authorities insisted on segregation. Accordingly racial residential segregation was mandated as official policy throughout all British colonies in tropical Africa. In 1912, metropolitan-based colonial authorities drew up a plan whose goal was to complete the racial segregation of all towns in these colonies within a period of ten years. They were not quite successful in their bid to segregate the older towns of Ghana such as Accra and Kumasi. However, they achieved considerable success in this regard with the newer towns. Curtin (1985) speculates that the relative ease of shaping the spatial pattern of a new town as opposed to existing ones, is one reason why despite the odds, colonial authorities were able to implement a racially segregated town plan for Tamale. At the time Tamale was the new capital of the Northern Territories of the Gold Coast. As a site for European colonial residential and administrative facilities, Tamale shared a lot of characteristics with sites that were typically selected for colonial government business. For one thing, it was located on a plateau. For another, it was situated a considerable distance away from the nearest native settlement. For yet another reason, it was surrounded by open space. Although Tamale provided the officials a clean slate to work with, they nevertheless, had to wrestle with a number of seemingly intractable problems. Prominent in this connection was the problem of protecting members of the European population from the Africans they came in contact with. One pragmatic solution was to isolate the entire colonial government staff from the native population at large. Another was to segregate the European from the African staff. Both propositions turned out to be expensive and served to bolster the case against segregation efforts.

Apart from Gambia, the Gold Coast (present-day, Ghana), and Sierra Leone, Britain controlled two other colonies in West Africa before World War I. These two colonies, Northern Nigeria and Southern Nigeria, were later merged to constitute the colony of Nigeria in 1914. These were the heydays of efforts to make tropical Africa a healthier place for Europeans to live and conduct private or colonial business. The colony of Southern Nigeria had a governor with medical expertise by the name of William MacGregor. He was intimately familiar with the medical findings and reports on malaria and other diseases that threatened the health of Europeans in the region. He was also aware of, but questioned, the recommendations of authorities in the Colonial Office in London. These authorities had recommended segregation as a means to achieve the goal of a healthier tropical Africa for Europeans. He was particularly troubled by the recommendation that parts of existing cities such as Lagos be demolished to create sanitary cordons as a health promotion strategy. In his opinion, such a move was tantamount to bad politics. The move, MacGregor, argued, would be violently opposed by members of the indigenous population. Furthermore, he believed, the strategy had a slim, if any, chance of succeeding. MacGregor was right, especially in view of the fact that violence broke out in Lagos in 1907. The violence was in opposition to a proposed sanitary segregation plan. The plan was to convert seven acres of urban land along the Lagos racecourse into a segregated European residential area. The land in question, it bears noting, had been confiscated from members of the native population. However, members of this population, supported by a number of other organized groups, particularly the Aborigines Protection Society were successful in thwarting this plan.

Governor MacGregor was steadfastly convinced that sanitary segregation was not a viable health promotion strategy. A successful and sustainable health promotion strategy, he believed, was one directed at attacking all threatening and potentially threatening diseases at their sources. In the case of malaria he argued as follows. If it could be concretely established that Africans were the reservoir for the parasites causing this life-threatening disease, it follows that eradicating it would entail focusing attention on Africans themselves. If anything, he went on, sanitary segregation could serve as no more than a temporary measure to control the spread of the disease.

Thus, Governor MacGregor broke ranks with most of his contemporaries in other colonies with respect to public health policy. In this connection, he instituted prophylactic measures such as the following: 1) requiring that all colonial government officials take quinine; 2) the gratis provision of quinine to everyone, including Africans, resident in Lagos and its suburbs; 3) the screening of all European residential units, offices and workplaces; and 4) the execution of regular campaigns to educate the public on methods to free their surroundings of mosquitoes.

Sir Frederick Lugard, the governor of the colony of Northern Nigeria, unlike MacGregor, subscribed to theories advocating racial residential segregation. In fact, Lugard was at the forefront of efforts to racially segregate the colonies. For him, segregation was more than a viable strategy for protecting the health of Europeans in Tropical Africa. Rather, it was a sound colonial governance tool. Conceivably, social control was easier in populations that are grouped by race than otherwise. Lugard had the entire territory of Northern Nigeria to test the tenability of theories extolling segregation as a public health or colonial governance tool. One of Lugard's first major actions in this regard was to replicate the cantonment system that had been implemented in British colonial India. In practice, this entailed relocating the administrative headquarters of Northern Nigeria from Lokoja to a new isolated site one mile (1.06km) away. Apart from adopting the cantonment system, Lugard adhered stringently to the Colonial Office's directives regarding racial segregation. Here, he issued edicts requiring the segregation of all district headquarters, including residential units or "rest houses" that served to accommodate exclusively European colonial government officials on tour away from the administrative headquarters. As a requirement, each of these units was located at least four hundred yards away from the closest residence of an African. This distance was not arbitrarily established. Rather, it was presumed to be a distance that could not be traversed by an Anopheles mosquito (*The Economist*, 1990).

Ironically, Africans who worked as domestic servants were allowed to live in servants' quarters in the European residential areas. Some have explained this irony as resulting from a desire on the part of Europeans "to be segregated but not inconvenienced" (Curtin, 1985: 605). Lugard was also persuaded by theories that linked health to environmental conditions as well as to physical activity. Accordingly, he sought to adopt construction policies based on, albeit antiquated scientific knowledge. For instance he recommended raising buildings on piers. This was believed to be an effective means of protecting buildings from having direct contact with tropical Africa's contaminated soil. Additionally, he set aside colonial government funds to provide or subsidize the provision of tennis courts, polo clubs, gulf courses and other recreational facilities. The aim was to encourage exercise through sporting activities amongst Europeans in Africa as a means of improving their health. If nothing else, Lugard deserves praise for his foresightedness in this regard. More than a century subsequent to his physical planning proposals, the world is awakening to the reality that spatial structures do indeed influence physical activity hence, human health. This is attested to by the plethora of recent works that have focused on the impact of the built environment on physical activity (see e.g., Frumkin, 2005; TRB, 2005; Hancock and Duhl, 1988). Lugard also subscribed to the notion that human health could be vastly improved by providing housing units with large verandahs and ample ventilation as well as protection against the units from direct rays from the sun.

Lugard's administration was bolder in its enactment and implementation of policies designed to accomplish public health objectives through the spatial segregation of the races than most others in the region. In this regard, the administration's chief authority on public health, Dr. M. Cameron, the Senior Sanitary Officer (for Northern Nigeria), proposed the enforcement of sanitary segregation laws in commercial areas as well. In practice, this meant that only Europeans were to own stores in these areas. In addition, no servants were to pass the night in the commercial districts. Lugard's town planning and public health policies resulted in a unique urban spatial structure in Northern Nigeria. A notable feature of this structure was the division into four distinct districts of each urban area born of European town planning efforts in the colony. The four districts were as follows (Njoh, 2008; Curtin, 1985): the colonial administrative and European residential district, located at least four hundred yards windward of all other areas; the commercial/industrial zone, located along the railway/station; the African clerks and high-ranking artisans' quarters; and the strangers' Quarters (or in Hausa, *Sabon Gari*). This latter serves as the home for native labourers and other less privileged members of the population. In the older urban settings such as Zaria and Kano, the *Sabon Gari* served as the residential areas for immigrants and not necessarily the underprivileged members of society. However, this group could most likely be found in *Sabon Gari* than any other part of town.

As time went by, protecting the health of Europeans through racial residential segregation increasingly gained ground as official policy throughout Northern Nigeria. At the same time the policy was gaining more and more support from members of the colonial medical community. In fact, this community is on record for approving the insertion in the *West African Pocket Book*—an informational manual for Europeans in West Africa—a passage claiming that racial segregation constitutes one of the most viable strategies for protecting Europeans against tropical diseases. In 1914, seven years after this, Lugard became Governor-General of Nigeria, which at this time had become a single colony. He immediately proceeded to make racial residential segregation the official government policy of colonial Nigeria. He was very forceful in this regard. Under the Township Ordinance of 1917, it was a crime punishable by a fine or imprisonment for any European to live in a non-European district.

The British were not the only colonial authorities who employed town planning schemes as a strategy for promoting public health. Rather, this strategy had become commonplace during the heydays of European colonialism in Africa (Njoh, 2008). Here, in contrast to other colonized regions such as India, colonial authorities had become more specific in stipulating segregation strategies. For instance, they specified the altitudes and linear distances from indigenous settlements that were necessary to promote the health of Europeans in the colonies. However, opinion varied widely with respect to the exact altitude and distances that were necessary to attain this objective. For example, while in some circles it was believed that an altitude of four hundred feet was sufficient, in others, the recommended altitude was three to five thousand feet (Curtin, 1985: 595). In tropical Africa, altitudes of five thousand feet were considered sufficient for safety once the anopheles mosquito had been identified as the vector for malaria. This is because five thousand feet was considered to be above the flight range of the mosquito. The decision of German colonial authorities to locate the administrative capital of colonial Cameroon (Kamerun) on the slopes of Mount Cameroon, which has an altitude of more than thirteen thousand feet (about 1,470m) was rooted in this belief.

The Germans were initially persuaded by theories advocating prophylactic measures such as the mass distribution of quinine as a means of protecting Europeans against tropical diseases. However, they later subscribed to the notion of sanitary segregation. In leaning towards sanitary segregation, a good number of German medical authorities argued that prophylactic measures such as mass 'quininization' were both impractical and infeasible. One reason for this was, these authorities argued, the fact that Africans were incapable of practicing proper mosquito control. Thus, they insisted on absolute segregation, which in some cases entailed the mass relocation of members of the native population to make room for "White Only" settlements. This was the case in Douala, Cameroon (Curtin, 1985: 6006). Here, German colonial officials had reached the rather dubious and baseless conclusion that as much as 72 per cent of the native population that was located along the city's seafront area was infested with the malaria parasite. This conclusion then constituted the basis of the decision to relocate all twenty thousand of the native residents of this area to an inland location. This case stands out in the annals of European colonial history for two main reasons. First the decision was indefensible on all logical grounds. Some credence to this assertion resides in the fact that members of the native population, European missionary and other philanthropic organizations in the colony vehemently opposed the decision. Also and paradoxically, members of the German colonial medical community who had advanced the notion of sanitary segregation went on record to assert that the decision made no sense on medical grounds. The opposition notwithstanding, the German colonial government in Cameroon, backed by their superiors in Berlin, pushed forward with the decision. The case is also noteworthy because of the ruthless manner in which the German colonial government reacted to the indigenous leadership's opposition to its indefensible decision. Some details on the nature of the opposition and said reaction are in order.

The native leadership of Douala had sought to oppose what it saw as the German colonial government's unjust decisions. This opposition was similar to others that had been waged by leaders of the native population in British colonies such as Ghana, Gambia and Nigeria. In Kamerun, German-educated King Rudolf Manga Bell, the indigenous leader of Douala, decided to petition the colonial government's decision to forcefully re-locate Africans. When the local colonial government ignored his petition, he proceeded, with the assistance of a German lawyer, to present his case, or more appropriately, the Douala people's case, to the *Kolonialamt* in Berlin and onward to the Reichstag. Upon noticing King Bell's persistence, the German colonial government in Kamerun decided to withdraw its recognition of him as the official leader of the people of Douala. On his part, King Bell decided to seek the support of other European powers in his bid to reclaim the ancestral lands of the Douala people that had been confiscated on the pretext of promoting public health by the German colonial authorities. This move on King Bell's part was made in summer 1914. This was the eve of World War I—a period that was marked by bitter tension and rivalry amongst Europeans. Once the war started, the German proceeded immediately to arrest King Bell and his secretary, Ngoso Din on the ridiculous and perfidious charge of treason. Both were tried, found guilty and executed by the German colonial government. The tragic conclusion to this tale cannot but make one to ponder the extent to which confiscating the seafront land of the Douala people was simply a strategy to protect the health of the town's European residents. Similar attempts at relocating native populations en masse in other parts of colonial Africa suggest that such policies sought to accomplish much more than public health goals. For instance, at one time during the heydays of British colonialism in East Africa, when the European population on Mombasa islands was only a mere 148 in comparison to 27,000 natives, a colonial medical officer had suggested that all natives be relocated to a location far-removed from the island (Curtin, 1985: 611).

Efforts to promote public health especially with respect to protecting the health of Europeans in French colonial Africa were informed by knowledge gleaned from the British colonial medical experience and experiments, especially those relating to mosquito/malaria control in the region. In fact, as far back as 1903, as Curtin (1985: 610) notes, "the standard French text of tropical hygiene had picked up the recent works of British antimalarial segregationists like Christopher and Stephens and presented them as the teachings of 'science.'" However, mosquitoes and malaria were not the only problems of concern to health authorities in colonial Africa. Other health problems included, but were by no means limited to, smallpox, whooping cough, tuberculosis, and plagues. Examples of this latter included the infamous bubonic plague that affected most of the continent between 1898 and 1914. The strategies designed to deal with contagious diseases and plagues such as this by French colonial authorities are worthy of note. This is particularly because of their spatial emphases. Apart from their inclination towards older ideas about controlling such diseases through quarantine, especially by creating *cordon sanitaires*, the French simply reversed the procedures to control malaria, which advocated the removal of Europeans from native areas. In contrast, they devised strategies requiring that infected natives be removed from European towns.

French architecture and urban planning made the task of distinguishing European from native towns quite easy. The French, perhaps more so than other Europeans, are well known for their efforts to create replicas of French towns in their colonial territories. The ancient city of Saint Louis (part of present-day Dakar), Senegal, was designed to take the form of an eighteenth century French town, complete with a central place, a gridiron street pattern and European-style buildings. From the onset, Saint Louis, which began having African mayors as far back as the eighteenth century, was never racially segregated. However, the newer City of Dakar, developed during a period of heightened racism in colonial Africa, was. Additionally, the French colonial authorities did everything possible, without portraying themselves as blatantly racist, to exclude members of the native population from Dakar. In this regard, and once again, under the pretext of protecting public health, they designated the most desirable section of the city as a "hygienic village." No traditional African structure, including all buildings of earth and thatch, was permitted in this section of the city. Under the same pretext, a zone containing no man-made structure—a sanitary cordon or *cordon sanitaire*—encircled the highest point in the city or the *plateau*. The *plateau* contained the residential units of Europeans. Elsewhere in francophone Africa, sanitary cordons were also used as a means to protect the health of the resident European population during the colonial era. For instance, in the Belgian Congo (present-day, Democratic Republic of Congo, formerly Zaire), Kalina, the European district, was separated from the rest of Leopoldville (now, Kinshasa) by a *cordon sanit*aire comprising a golf course, a botanical garden, and a zoo. Members of the native population, with the exception of domestic servants, were not permitted in Kalina from 9 p.m. to 6 a.m. Africans were allowed in the area only during these hours under exceptional circumstances such as emergencies. Also, no Europeans were permitted in the native areas during same hours.

In 1914, when the bubonic plague was visited upon the city of Dakar, the French colonial government immediately ordered the burning of all traditional housing units as well as all the units in which any plague victim lived around European districts. This measure, the colonial authorities argued, was needed to protect the health of Europeans in the city. The colonial government further ordered the mass relocation of the remainder of the native population to a new African town on the periphery of the city. The new town was christened Medina after identical towns in North Africa. All accounted for, some thirty-eight thousand Africans were relocated in the process (Curtin, 1985: 12).

Members of the native population were, as their counterparts in the case of Douala, Accra, Barthurst, Freetown and Lagos, opposed to any form of relocation, let alone mass relocation. However, their opposition was tempered by the fact that the policy was sold as one designed to protect their own health. It is important to note that in 1914, Dakar and a number of other communes in Senegal were successful in electing their own native representatives to the National Assembly in Paris. With the presence of Africans in the French National Assembly, it became increasingly difficult for French authorities to enact any blatantly racist policies on public health or any other false pretext. Thus, they resorted to policies that discriminated on the basis of culture as opposed to race. Hence, while a distinct European town continued to exist, its distinguishing features were in terms of architectural style as opposed to its racial composition. In fact, it was possible for anyone to live in a European town as long as he or she was prepared to abide by European standards of architecture and social behaviour.

# Chapter 4

# Racism Versus Health Concerns as the Rationale for Racial Segregation

## Introduction

Efforts to identify the rationale for racial residential segregation policies in colonial Africa have left much to be desired. Analysts are wont to identify non-controversial factors such as the outbreak of epidemics and/or the prevalence of malaria as the justification for these policies (Home, 1997; Christopher, 1991; 1983; Goerg, 1987; Curtin, 1985; Gale, 1980). Yet, there is a preponderance of evidence suggesting that the European proclivity for racially segregating populations predated: 1) recorded major outbreaks of epidemics in multi-racial settings anywhere in the world; and 2) the discovery in West Africa of the anopheles mosquito as the vector of the malaria parasite.

This chapter deviates from the norm by identifying the ideology of race as the motivating factor behind racial spatial segregation schemes in colonial Africa. Thus, the chapter refutes arguments portraying racial residential segregation as a strategy for promoting and/or protecting health. The race ideology successfully dehumanized Africans while affirming the imagined superiority of Europeans especially in the early-nineteenth century. The chapter contends that racial residential segregation policies in colonial Africa were a function of the race ideology that dominated the discourse on human relations in the West in the early-nineteenth century. An important criterion for establishing causality in social science is that the alleged cause must chronologically precede the observed effect (see e.g., Babbie, 2004). Accordingly, the chapter presents evidence to demonstrate that racial residential segregation did not become official policy in colonial Africa until the publication of pseudo-scientific works purporting to lend credence to the prevailing race ideology of the time.

The chapter begins in the next section by discussing the ideology of race in European ethos. Following this, is a discussion of European colonial racial residential segregation initiatives in Africa. Next, the chapter presents a sample of cases of colonial racial residential segregation schemes from all major regions of the continent, including the North, West, Central, East and Southern Africa. A subsequent section discusses the cases with a view to showing how colonial racial residential segregation policies were shaped not by the need to promote public health but by the race ideology of the time. The chapter concludes by highlighting the implications of these policies for contemporary development initiatives in Africa.

## The ideology of race in western ethos

Race is an ideology and not a scientific concept or an element of human biology. As an ideology, 'racial classification' has been employed to justify the differential treatment of people based on the meanings attributed to their varying physical characteristics. To the extent that race is a social as opposed to a biological construct, it arose historically. An appreciation of this history is important in the context of this discussion. It can help explain the urban planning schemes that European colonial powers crafted to institute racial spatial segregation structures in Africa. The ideology of race developed especially in Western Europe and Northern America in the period leading up to the onset of the formal European colonial era in Africa (circa, 1884). It has its roots in the enslavement of Africans in the Americas dating as far back as the fifteenth century. Certainly, slavery cannot be meaningfully tied to skin colour. However, the race ideology and concomitant dehumanization of people of African heritage has everything to do with their skin colour and cognate physical characteristics.

Africans were neither the first nor the only group ever enslaved. The annals of human history dating back to biblical times contain rich accounts of the institution of slavery. In Europe, ancient Greeks, Romans, and other groups legitimized the institution of slavery. The English are on record for enslaving their Irish brethrens. In fact, the English had enslaved the Irish to work on plantations in the Americas long before people of African origin became the slaves of choice for this task. The law in Tudor England allowed for the enslavement of vagabonds. By some accounts, the Irish and Indians outnumbered people of African origin as slaves on English plantations during the earlier phase of large-scale plantation agriculture in Barbados and Jamaica (Smedley, 1993).

True as the foregoing accounts are, it is foolhardy and indeed insincere to trivialize the role of physical characteristics in the construction of the race ideology. Some have pointed to these examples as proof that the ideology of race and the concomitant dehumanization of people of African origin have nothing to do with their peculiar 'African features,' particularly their dark skin. For instance, Barbara Fields has argued that White slaves were as brutally treated by their (White) masters as Black slaves (Fields, 1990; 1982). "The English," she contended, "considered no brutality too extreme in bringing to heel the supposedly savage and undoubtedly fair skinned Irish" (Fields, 1990: 102-102). Fields and other like-minded analysts contend that the race ideology is all about slavery. It is not. The ideology of race within the context of the present discussion can be defined as follows (Nash, 1962: 285):

> A system of ideas which interprets and defines the meanings of racial differences, real or imagined, in terms of some system of cultural values. The ideology of race is always normative: it ranks differences as better or worse, superior or inferior, desirable or undesirable, and as modifiable or unmodifiable.

As demonstrated below, the race ideology, specifically designed to dehumanize people of African origin, is rooted in the slave history of Africans in Northern America. This must not be taken to mean that the ideology of race emerged simultaneously with the institution of slavery. Yet, it is not a quantum leap to contend that the slave status of people of African origins in the Americas facilitated the construction of the race ideology, which confers on these same people an inferior or less-than-human status. By the time the American Constitution was being crafted, the race ideology was still in its infancy. However, it must be noted that at that time the institution of slavery had evolved to the point where slave owners were wholly White while the enslaved were completely of African origin. In fact, by the seventeenth century, the enslavement of other than people of African origin had been outlawed in the US (Smedley, 1993). Therefore, when the US Constitution, in Article 1 Section 2, equates one "free person" to three other persons (read slaves), it was in fact equating one White person to three persons of African origin. Any alternative read or interpretation of the three-fifths clause in this Constitution as some have tried to do is inaccurate (see e.g., Fields, 1990). Efforts to disentangle the physical and other attributes of Africans vis-à-vis those of people of European descent from the race ideology discourse may be well-meaning but by all means misleading.

By the latter part of the seventeenth century two developments culminating in the further isolation of people of African origins had occurred (Smedley, 1993). The first was the astronomical growth in the demand for labour in the plantations of the so-called New World. People of African origin, it was believed, emerged as better suited than their Irish and Indian counterparts for the tedious task of plantation agriculture. Those who harboured this view also concluded that people of African origin were immune to old world diseases. The second development had to do with the real and potential threat to social order posed by poor freed White slaves who were persistently demanding lands and other privileges from the pro-upper class colonial government. At this point, the colonial authorities were unified in concluding that resorting to African labour served as a viable strategy to ward off any threats from poor Whites.

Another major event that served to further racialize slavery and in fact, energize the race ideology was the entry of Englishmen into the slave trade. The English public (at home) was not enthusiastic about this development. If for no other reason, it is because this development coincided with the era of the ideals of equality, justice, democracy and human rights in the evolution of Western political philosophy. To rationalize their actions, the slave traders deemed it necessary to dehumanize people of African origin. Africans, the English slave traders argued, were heathen and in darkness, and that it was a Christian duty to shine light upon them as well as save their souls.

Efforts to rationalize the institution of slavery were up against fierce opposition from a burgeoning anti-slavery movement in Europe and North America. By the end of the eighteenth century, pro-slavery forces were working tirelessly to build and buttress their case for slavery, particularly the enslavement of people of African origin. This led to a focus on what they considered the physical peculiarities of African people. From that point (mid-eighteenth century) on, pro-slavery and like-minded groups spared no opportunity to make their case. They stridently attempted, albeit unsuccessfully, to show how the physical and other real or imagined features of African people were unique, and invariably made them inferior to Europeans.

From the late-eighteenth century, the term race, its ambiguity notwithstanding, had risen to prominence in the lexicon of human socio-political discourse. In fact, its use for human classification purposes focused particularly on physical attributes. In practice, and as an ideology, racial classification effectively tied the socio-political status to the physical traits of individuals thereby creating a manufactured and novel form of social identity (Smedley, 1993). By the time of the American Revolution, pro-slavery groups had successfully formulated a new ideology, namely the race ideology (Davis, 1999). The classification system produced by this ideology grouped together all people of European descent, without regard to socio-economic status, into one group called, 'White.' The system placed people of African origin, regardless of socio-economic status, into another group also called, "Negro." This categorization scheme was ordinal. It arranged the two groups hierarchically such that Whites occupied the top-most rung, while Blacks occupied the lowest rung of the structure. The rest of humanity or other 'racial' groups were, within this racist framework, believed to occupy different rungs between these two extremes. As shown below, this hierarchical schema dictated not only the social status of groups, but also constituted the basis for apportioning society's resources to different groups. Proponents of slavery contended that the differential access to resources or other inequalities in life were, like the physical features of different groups, naturally predetermined. These deep-seated beliefs about the varying physical features of people originated from different geographical regions make the American version of slavery unique. In fact, as some have observed, the only system of slavery in the world that was 'racialized' (Davis, 1999; Smedley, 1993; Frederickson, 1988; Jordan, 1968).

By tying servitude to physical characteristics or so-called racial features, this invented classification system had conferred on people of African origin an inferior status vis-à-vis other groups, but particularly in relation to people of European origin. Although the fact that slaves were black while the masters were white was an accident of history, it nevertheless provided fodder for the rancorous debate on race in Europe, and the race theory it gave birth to in the eighteenth century (ICL, Online). Here, it must be noted that at the end of the eighteenth century the reigning ideology of race had transformed the slave who happened to be black and had been rendered socially inferior by virtue of being enslaved, "into a person who was inferior because he was black and hence fitted for slavery" (ICL, Online, para. 3). For the slave master, the enslaved was simply a chattel and anything but a human being (Fanon, 1967).

Slaves were supposed to be both persons and property or human beings and chattels (Smedley, 1993). This classification posed difficult problems for government authorities and slave owners in general. Which one of these rights comes or ought to come first? For the enslaved, it would have been preferable for their status as humans to be ranked higher than their status as property (of the slave owner). Yet, because of their connection to the levers of power, slave masters were able to ensure that the status of enslaved people as slaves ranked higher than their identity as persons. Thus, slave masters effectively downplayed or minimized those qualities that made enslaved people, humans. Evidence to the effect that slave owners succeeded in the goal of dehumanizing people of African origin abound. For instance, the US Constitution neither recognized the enslaved or what at the time was known as 'negroes,' as humans nor extended to them citizenship rights.

The mid-1800s, that is, the period immediately preceding the onset of the European colonial era in Africa, witnessed intensive efforts to provide scientific justification for the folk theory of 'White superiority' on the one hand, and 'Black inferiority' on the other. In the United States, scholars who subscribed to this theory strived to marshal every piece of evidence that could lend credence to the baseless belief that Africans were not only biologically different from Europeans but constituted a lower species of humans. In the 1830s, Samuel Morton (1799-1851) embarked on research in the field of so-called 'craniometry.' This turned out to be the first school of American anthropology, which supported the race ideology. Morton and others of his ilk measured the insides of crania, originating from many and diverse populations, with the aim of proving that the crania of Africans, hence their brains, were smaller than those of people of European descent. This, the 'scientists' argued, was proof positive that people of European origin were more intelligent than their African counterparts.

To be sure, efforts to reinforce the notion of 'White supremacy' were also taking place in Europe around this time. In France, for instance, Arthur Comte de Gobineau (1816-1882), who wrote a book, captioned *An Essay on the Inequality of Human Races*, earned the dubious title of 'father of modern racial demography' (see Gobineau, 1853). It is in this book that Gobineau developed his racist theory of the Aryan master race. The book advocated the notion that race created culture and argued that differences among people from Africa, Europe and Asia constituted natural barriers. He opposed 'race-mixing, which he believed would inevitably result in chaos. In 1854, George Gliddon, co-edited a book with the caption, *Types of Mankind*. The book rank-ordered all groups of humans and concluded that people of African origin were by nature, closer to apes than to humans.

Efforts to prove the imagined superiority of Europeans vis-à-vis 'racial others,' as futile as they were, constituted the basis of public policy designed to, among other things, maintain the purity of the so-called Aryan race. Racial residential segregation policies and laws that incriminated sexual relations between Europeans and 'racial others,' especially people of African origin, are rooted in the revelations of these pseudo-scientific works. While physical segregation was designed to serve as a symbol of unequal social statuses, miscegenation laws were designed to preserve the purity of the 'Caucasian race.' As Smedley (1993) noted:

From its inception separateness and inequality was what 'race' was all about. The attributes of inferior race status came to be applied to free blacks as well as slaves. In this way, 'race' was configured as an autonomous new mechanism of social differentiation that transcended the slave condition and persisted as a form of social identity long after slavery ended.

By 1884 when the European colonial era began in Africa (circa, 1880s), the notion of Africans as the 'inferior race' and Europeans as the 'superior race' was already crystallized and cemented in the minds of many. This notion constituted the basis for institutionalizing racial segregation through the infamous Jim Crow laws of the post-Civil War era in the US (circa, 1870s). Thus, it is herein submitted that racial spatial segregation policies that European colonial authorities adopted in Africa drew some modicum of inspiration from the Jim Crow laws, which on their part, were grounded in the racist beliefs and arguments of pro-slavery groups. It is no coincidence that European colonial powers employed verbatim the same arguments that had been advanced by these groups to justify the enslavement of people of African origin to rationalize the colonization of Africa. The European claim of either cultural or racial superiority is at the root of racial residential segregation policies that set aside the best sites for Europeans in colonial towns. The claim also constitutes the basis of public health programmes that sought to protect the health of Europeans while ignoring that of Africans during the colonial era.

**European colonialism and racially segregated spatial structures in Africa**

A common feature of colonial towns in Africa, from Dakar to Mogadishu and from Cairo to Cape Town, was their racially segregated spatial structure. However, it is important to note that racial segregation did not become official policy in the region until the 1900s subsequent to the development of the race ideology. As the selected cases from all major regions of the continent, viz., north, west, central, southern, and east/Indian Ocean, suggest, prior to the 1900s racial integration was the norm.

*North Africa*

Modernist urban planning activities did not occur at a significant level in North Africa until the onset of the nineteenth century. This is when the region fell under the socio-economic dominion of Europe, which increasingly shaped its domestic and international affairs. By the late-nineteenth century most parts of the region were already under the colonial or other form of politico-economic control of a European power. For example, the French were in effective control of Algeria (1830), Tunisia (1881), and Morocco (1912). On its part, Britain had won control over Egypt (1882) and Italy had taken control of Libya (1911). By 1914, the colonial and imperial tentacles of European powers had spread into every crevice of the region. These powers proceeded to rapidly modernize the region particularly as a way of getting back at the Ottoman Empire. The empire's suzerainty had extended to many parts of Europe for five centuries before the European conquest. In the area of urban planning this meant the widespread introduction of Western land, spatial organization principles and building materials and techniques.

The introduction of such principles in North Africa best illustrates the proclivity on the part of Europeans to affirm their perceived supremacy over 'racial others.' Here, it must be noted that the North African region has a history of urbanization complete with several well-developed and densely populated human settlements predating the European colonial era (UN-GRHS, 2009). For instance, the Arab city of Tunis, located about 15 kilometres from the ancient city of Carthage, was established as far back as the seventh century. As Finlay and Paddison (1986) have noted, cities such as Tunis were established, and served, as a centre of sacred Islamic religious, learning and cultural activities. The Islamic tendency to distinguish between public and private space dictated a need to build walls around these cities. European colonial authorities made hardly any effort to understand the nature and functioning of Islamic cities. Instead, they found the cities, or what the French called *les villes des indigènes*, unfit for habitation by Europeans. Many of the Europeans had decided to settle permanently in the region. Accordingly, they proceeded to develop European enclaves (or *les villes des Europeènes*), complete with broad, straight boulevards, European style buildings and concomitant amenities. In Tunis, the European city, which was completed in 1898, was located between the Bab Bhar and the port of Tunis (Finlay and Paddison, 1986).

In Morocco, French colonial authorities established European cities alongside the medinas but actively discouraged any meaningful interaction between them. There was a general tendency on the part of colonial urban planners in the region to replicate well known European urban designs such as Haussmann's design of Paris. At the same time, colonial development policies ensured the concentration of all modern social and economic activities in the European districts. Before long, the traditional Islamic districts had declined in importance as economic and administrative centres. In some cases, such as that of the Kasbah in Tunis, the Medinas were stripped of their enclosing walls (Finlay and Paddison, 1986). Throughout the region, the European enclaves stood in stark morphological economic and social contrast to the traditional Islamic towns or Medinas. The enclaves were designed to serve the exclusive interest of the European settler community. Thus, urban centres in the region functioned as two communities in one, where de facto racial segregation was the norm. Apart from spatial segregation, Brown (1973) noted that certain jobs were reserved for the Europeans and others for the natives. He further noted that, there was a level below which the European could not fall and a ceiling which marked the highest point to which a native could not rise (Ibid).

*West Africa*

The presence of Europeans in West Africa dates as far back as the fifteenth century. The Portuguese built Elmina Castle in Ghana in 1482 and by 1659, the French had set up a permanent outpost in St. Louis, Senegal. Up until the 1820s, it was not uncommon for European traders and their employees to share living facilities (Goerg, 1998; Gale, 1980; Betts, 1971). For example, in Freetown, Sierra Leone, British and wealthy Sierra Leoneans of Creole extraction were known to live in the same buildings. All of this changed in the late-1800s, when racial segregation policies were promulgated throughout the region.

One of the best known of these policies was adopted in Senegal in 1914. Between September and October of that year, some 2900 members of the native population were relocated from Dakar proper to constitute an exclusive African village on an undesirable piece of land to the north-west of the city (Betts, 1971). This decision to create an all-African village was reached during the tenure of Governor-General William Ponty. Officially, this policy was a reaction to the outbreak of a bubonic plague that occurred in the city beginning in April 1914. As part of the relocation efforts, all buildings of local or so-called sub-standard materials were destroyed. No new construction was permitted unless it was of European materials. In other words, only European-type buildings or what the French colonial authorities called, *construction à l'europeène* were permitted.

French colonial authorities were not unique in this regard. Earlier on in 1901 the British Colonial Office had made a decision to racially segregate all of its colonies in tropical Africa (Frenkel and Western, 1988). Three years prior to that, a medical team from the Liverpool School of Tropical Medicine under the leadership of Dr. Ronald Ross, had incriminated the anopheles mosquito as the vector of the malaria parasite. Members of the indigenous population, British colonial authorities had observed, were already infected with malaria while Europeans were not. Furthermore, the scientific observations of Ross and his collaborators revealed that anopheles mosquitoes were nocturnal as they transmitted the malaria-causing parasite uniquely at night. Based on these two observations, British colonial authorities mandated that Europeans could interact with members of the native population only during the day and must return to exclusive European residential areas at night. These authorities deemed such segregation necessary as a prophylaxis against malaria for members of the resident European population. The first major project that was meant to transform this policy into reality was implemented in Sierra Leone. Here, British colonial authorities constructed an exclusive European enclave, the Hill Station, in 1904. The enclave reposes on a hill overlooking, and linked to, Freetown by a custom-built 'mountain railway.' Malaria was by no means the only disease whose potential to spread was used by British colonial authorities as a pretext for adopting racial spatial segregation policies in West Africa. In Ghana, the outbreak of the bubonic plague and yellow fever epidemics in 1908 and 1910 was employed as a pretext for racially segregating Accra and Kumasi (Gale, 1980).

*Central Africa*

The French, who controlled most of the Central African region during the colonial era were also inclined to adopt racial spatial segregation policies. This is paradoxical given that the French always denied being racist. Yet, in Africa, the French went beyond creating exclusive enclaves for Europeans to promulgating legislation designed to limit the expression of African tradition and culture. In this regard, French colonial authorities in Brazzaville enacted a decree in 1904 that restricted the playing of drums, dancing and other merrymaking activities by Africans to certain hours and days of the week (Martin, 1995). According to the decree such activities were authorized only once a week from 6 pm on Saturday until Sunday morning. Five years subsequent to this, the authorities promulgated a law that created two 'native-only' neighbourhoods, namely Bacongo and Poto-Poto, in a swampy area at the outskirts of Brazzaville (Ibid). One provision of the law was a curfew that required members of the native population not to be out of their homes after 9pm. Across the Congo River Belgian colonial authorities had established similar policies in Leopoldville (present-day Kinshasa). Here, there were also curfews (9pm–4am) and segregated neighbourhoods for Africans.

*Southern Africa*

In colonial Zimbabwe, authorities had developed an elaborate scheme, which classified the colony's races into three hierarchically arranged categories with Europeans occupying the highest point, followed by Asians and/or 'coloured people' and the Blacks or indigenous Africans at the bottom. Town planning laws were designed to protect the health of the people according to this pecking order. In the case of Ndola, one of colonial Zimbabwe's local municipalities, White residential areas were generously furnished with sanitary amenities, including in-door toilets, large residential units, gardens, well-maintained lighted streets and so on. In contrast, the indigenous African neighbourhoods boasted hardly any sanitation facilities. In the mid-1930s, the indigenous African neighbourhood in Ndola, which comprised as many as 4,000 people, was provided with only 1,700 mud huts, as few as fifty pit latrines and no other sanitary facility.

South Africa stands out among African countries for its apartheid policy that was in force until the mid-1990s when the country became democratic. The roots of the country's first official policies designed to specifically separate Whites from "racial others" have been traced by some to East London (Maylam, 1995). Here, racial segregation became official policy in 1849. This is when the government mandated the spatial segregation of 'Fingoes and other so-called coloured natives' from the Whites. Almost a decade later in 1857, a law designed to control members of the indigenous population in the town's 'Native Village' was enacted. By 1872, East London had already earned the dubious reputation of 'a town with clear legacy of enforced racial separation' (Maylam, 1995). By the mid-nineteenth century, other Eastern Cape towns, including Cradock, Graaf-

Reinet, and Grahamstown had adopted urban racial segregation as official policy. These policies were precursors to the country's nation-wide apartheid laws. Two of the most prominent in this regard are the Natives Land Act No. 27 of 1913 and the Natives (Urban Areas) Act of 1923. These laws were designed to limit the access of non-Whites to urban and other highly desirable areas.

*East Africa and the Indian Ocean region*

As argued above, the prevailing European philosophy on race during the colonial era elevated Europeans far above 'racial others.' This philosophy was accorded real meaning in Africa by the racial distribution of urban space that culminated in Europeans occupying not only the largest but also the most highly desirable parcels of land. For instance, in colonial Kenya, Nairobi's 'racial tripartition' resulted in the following racial spatial segregation structure (K'Akumu and Olima, 2007). The entire picturesque north-western areas, which contained the city's most valuable land was designated as an exclusive European enclave. The second-best desirable areas in the city's north-eastern region were assigned to Asians. Members of the native population were assigned the small and least desirable area in the eastern and southern quadrant of the city.

In Madagascar, French colonial authorities under the auspices of the island's pioneer colonial governor, General Gallieni (beginning in 1896), took a number policy actions relating to urban planning that can be reasonably interpreted as racist. For instance, neither the planning commission that was appointed by Gallieni in 1896 nor the one that was established more than two decades later included an indigenous African member (Njoh, 2008). Also, Gallieni's appointee to design the island's major towns, Georges Cassaigne, was avowedly in favour of racial spatial segregation. Furthermore, Gallieni's successor, Marcel Olivier, was also a proponent of segregation. In fact, Olivier contended that the segregation of 'native' districts is indispensable in colonial cities and should not be construed as constituting racial discrimination (Njoh, 2008; Wright, 1991). The crux of his argument is that the type of segregation he advocated was based not on race but on living standard. In 1928, the governor-general took action to establish zones in which only 'European construction' was authorized. This policy was essentially a replica of the one that had been promulgated by Governor-General William Ponty two decades earlier in Senegal. French colonial authorities believed that their spatial policies had no racist objectives. Rather, they argued that the policies were designed to simply promote European living standards. In an interview for the *Tribune de Madagascar* in 1924, for instance, architect Georges Cassaigne is quoted as explicitly condoning segregation for "those who cannot or will not live by European standards" (Wright, 1991: 278). The group Cassaigne was bent on privileging included the White proletariat of the colony.

## Race ideology, health and spatial policies in colonial Africa

The conventional justifications for the policy of racial spatial segregation in Africa have been given to typically include the following: 1) the 'natural tendency for humans to congregate based on certain shared attributes;' (Fields, 1990) 2) a practice that had occurred in medieval Europe more than five centuries before the European colonial era began in Africa (Christopher, 1983); 3) the need to preserve and protect European culture (Wright, 1991); and 4) the need to protect the health of Europeans (Goerg, 1998). The remainder of this chapter is dedicated to interrogating these rationales for racial segregation. The ultimate aim is to demonstrate that none of these justifications is as persuasive as the ideology of race in explaining the racial spatial segregation policies that were adopted by European colonial authorities throughout Africa.

*The 'natural tendency hypothesis.'*

The question of centrality in this chapter is not about why or how these two groups (Europeans and Africans) came together. Rather, it is about the policies that Europeans in their capacity as rulers enacted to govern the larger space (i.e., towns) within which they and the 'ruled' co-existed. As shown above, racial spatial segregation was the rule and not the exception throughout colonial Africa. Barbara Fields (e.g., 1990) and like-minded analysts attribute such spatial structures to the so-called natural tendency of humans to live in close proximity with those they share major features such as language, skin colour, heritage and so on. This theory suggests that colonial Africa's racially segregated spatial structures resulted from a preference for segregation rather than integration on the part of Africans as well as Europeans. Empirical evidence does not lend support to this theory. Rather, the racial spatial segregation policies that were adopted throughout colonial Africa were inspired by the ideology of race that had developed in Europe during the eighteenth to nineteenth centuries.

Before the race ideology gained prominence, Europeans in Africa had no problem sharing living space with Africans. As Goerg (1998) and Gale (1980) have noted, this was as true in British colonies as it was in the French ones. For example, Europeans and wealthy Africans in Freetown in British colonial Sierra Leone not only shared the same life style but lived in the same districts. In the early-1800s, it was commonplace to find a two-storey house with one of its floors occupied by a European tenant and the other by its African owner. Similarly, in Saint Louis in French colonial Senegal, French traders and their African agents and employees did not only share living districts but also shared buildings in some cases (Bonnardel, 1992; Gale, 1980). Instances of co-habitation such as the afore-cited render hollow any hypothesis postulating that racially segregated spatial structures in colonial Africa were a function of the desire on the part of members of different racial groups to live exclusively with 'their own kind.'

A stronger case against such a hypothesis resides in the fact that Africans vehemently challenged the policy of racial spatial segregation throughout the continent. In fact, as Thomas Gale (1980) noted, no feature of the colonial enterprise was as resented as the policy of segregation. A policy initiative by Governor Walter Egerton of colonial Southern Nigeria, which culminated in the ejection of 350 Africans from prime land in Lagos provoked a barrage of petitions from the civil society, local elites, and the press. As Gale (1980) revealed, even a member of the British Parliament in London is on record for opposing racial segregation policies in British colonial Africa. In Freetown, as noted in the previous chapter, the existence of a professional class of Africans, including doctors, lawyers and accountants, predated the formal onset of the colonial era in 1884. It is therefore no wonder that the decision to create an exclusive European enclave was also fiercely protested in Freetown. Among the many reasons for this resentment is the fact that the creation of exclusive European enclaves required the investment of funds generated by heavily taxing members of the native population. Further opposition to such enclaves was rooted in the fact their creation, in some cases, required not only the re-location of upper class Africans from prime land but also the concomitant neglect of so-called native towns. While the resistance was largely peaceful, there were instances involving violence. Instances of this latter genre were recorded throughout the continent in towns as far apart as Dakar, Senegal (Gale, 1980), Freetown, Sierra Leone (Goerg, 1998), Brazzaville, Congo (PR) (Martin, 1995), and Antsinarabe, Madagascar (Wright, 1991).

*The 'European medieval origins hypothesis.'*

Some analysts have traced the origins of racial spatial segregation policies in Africa not to the ideology of race but to the medieval era in Europe. For instance, Christopher contends that the British policy of racial segregation in colonial South Africa has its roots in the early English colonization of Wales and Ireland (Christopher, 1983). Thus, Christopher locates the origins of the policy in the spatial organization policies that were promulgated by King Edward I in the thirteenth century at Flint, Conway and Caernarvon (Ibid, p. 145). In an attempt to lend further credence to the 'colonial origin hypothesis,' Christopher contends that, British colonial and imperial authorities have been consistent in their resistance to the integration of differing cultural groups.

The hypothesis can be challenged on two crucial grounds. First, the claim of consistency on the part of the British is not credible. In fact, racial spatial segregation did not become official policy in British colonies until later on during the colonial époque in Africa (see below). Prior to that, as stated earlier, British and other Europeans lived in the same districts and in some cases, in the same facilities with Africans. Second, the fact that the British in Wales and Ireland lived apart from the natives did not result from some official policy. Rather, it was a product of the constant hostilities of the natives towards the British who were viewed and treated as invaders. On the contrary, Africans generally welcomed Europeans—a gesture that some Europeans were quick to characterize as indicative of docility. The Governor-General of colonial Senegal, William Ponty employed this characterization in a telegraph to the French Minister of the Colonies expressing his pleasant surprise at the lack of resistance to French colonial policies. In the telegraph dated 30 August, 1914, the governor stated thus, the "entire population complies with the greatest docility to all measures taken … " (Betts, 1971: 145).

At any rate, it is worth reiterating, that the policy of racial spatial segregation was preceded by a practice of racial integration and even co-habitation. This was the case throughout colonial Africa. The situation involving French as well as British colonial West Africa has already been alluded to. In South Africa, the Dutch had established racially integrated spatial structures. These structures, as Nuttall noted, were deemed chaotic by the British who subscribed to the 19th century race ideology that promoted the notion of European racial superiority and advocated the need to preserve 'Aryan racial purity' (Nutall, 2004). Consequently they (the British) moved speedily to create racially segregated spatial structures.

*The 'preservation of European culture hypothesis.'*

A perusal of European colonial and imperial ventures reveals the existence of two major overlapping premises for discrimination against 'racial others.' One is racial and the other is socio-cultural. These two premises reflect two major philosophies, namely Eurocentrism and the Enlightenment theories of universalism (Goerg, 1998). Conventional wisdom attributes the tendency to emphasize culture as the distinguishing mark between Europeans and 'racial others' to the French. This is erroneous as Europeans of all origins had the tendency to use culture as a basis for discriminating against 'racial others.' The fact that the British were just as likely as the French to deride African culture and employ this latter as a basis for adopting racial segregation policies lends credence to this assertion. In Conakry and Brazzaville, as noted above, the French viewed with disdain African cultural and traditional practices such as singing and drumming. At the same time they believed that European culture was under threat from African and other cultures. These two reasons served as the basis for adopting the policy of racial spatial segregation in colonial towns. For instance, a French colonial authority is quoted as contending that such segregation was necessary in Conakry for the following reason. Segregation provided members of the native population with an exclusive enclave in which they could shout and beat their drums as loudly as they wanted, as well as dance for as long as they desired (Goerg, 1998). This paternalistic rationalization of segregation thinly veils the racist proclivities of Europeans of the time. On their part, British colonial authorities rationalized their racial segregation policies by arguing that Africans were too noisy for their liking. One colonial official was quoted as stating thus (Goerg, 1998: 11):

The good people in this country do not seem to know that noise is objectionable. They are born in noise, live in noise, die in noise, and cannot realize that noise is unpleasant to anybody.

It is easy to appreciate the fact that the cultural difference was only a pretext to adopt segregation policies in Africa. Here, it bears drawing attention to the fact that segregation was the rule even in colonial towns such as Freetown, where a significant number of Africans were descendants of formerly enslaved Africans in Britain and Nova Scotia. Thus, although these 'Europeanized' Africans shared the same values and culture with Europeans, they were never accepted in the exclusive European enclaves.

*The 'European health protection hypothesis.'*

The relevant literature is dominated by works that identify the need to protect the health of Europeans as the *raison d'être* for racial spatial segregation policies throughout colonial Africa. In an otherwise balanced portrayal of the evolution of this policy in British West Africa, Thomas Gale (1980) appeared to be persuaded by the rhetoric of colonial authorities when he made the following statement with respect to the policy to segregate Accra and Kumasi in colonial Ghana:

It [i.e., racial segregation] might not have become the general policy after 1910 if it had not been for certain unprecedented developments—the outbreaks of plague and yellow fever epidemics in 1908 and 1910—which alarmed the medical authorities into recommending residential segregation as being absolutely essential to the protection of the lives of the European officials (p. 496).

On her part, Ordile Goerg (1998) recounts the events that led to the adoption of racial segregation as official policy in colonial Africa. According to Goerg, the incrimination of the anopheles mosquito as the vector of the malaria causing parasite explains why Joseph Chamberlain, the British Secretary of State for the Colonies (1895–1903) mandated racial spatial segregation in the colonies. Segregation from the natives, Chamberlain argued, was the only promising strategy for protecting Europeans from malarial infection in Africa (Ibid).

The foregoing and similar accounts are misleading. The position of this chapter is that segregation policies would have been promulgated even without the outbreaks of any epidemic. Thus, the promotion or protection of health was only a pretext and not the veritable reason for racial segregation policies. A close reading of the confidential British correspondences of the colonial era by Frenkel and Western (1988) revealed that segregation was conditioned by the pervasive racial thinking of the time, rather than a concern for the health of Europeans. The pervasive racial thinking held that Europeans were superior to, and that their lives were worth more than those of, Africans. Witness for instance, the fact that colonial authorities sought to protect the health of European officials while ignoring that of Africans.

Other inconsistencies in the colonial residential and spatial organization policies of the time also suggest that racial segregation was intended to accomplish goals that had very little if anything to do with protecting the health of Europeans. In this regard, it is necessary to note that in theory, protecting Europeans from malaria required nocturnal segregation. However, in practice, many Africans, including domestic servants and mistresses or concubines of Europeans lived in so-called exclusive European enclaves. In fact, each bungalow in Hill Station, Freetown, for instance, was provided with housing for one-to-two domestic servants (Goerg, 1998). These inconsistencies alone are not enough as a reason to conclude that racial segregation, particularly the creation of exclusive European enclaves, was a function of the pervasive racial thinking of the time as opposed to a concern for public health. Rather, this conclusion can be easily arrived at by paying some attention to the discourse on the race question especially in the United States and Western Europe during the heydays of colonialism in Africa.

Pejorative and derisive characterizations of Africans were commonplace in intellectual and political circles in Western Europe and the United States at the time. For example, Ronald Ross, who is best known in the annals of British colonial history for his role in identifying the anopheles mosquito as the vector of malaria is said to have once characterized Africans as follows. They are child-like and "somewhat like black Irish; merry, full of life, and extraordinarily musical" (Goerg, 1998: 224). Similarly, confidential correspondences between colonial officials on the ground in Africa and their superiors and others in their home countries contained characterizations of Africans that were by all measures racist. One such correspondence, viewed the unsanitary conditions of African towns as a function of Africans being "unable to keep a clean city" and "too lazy to look after their own comfort" (Goerg, 1998). The theory of segregation as a public health policy is rendered even more tenuous by the fact that some European colonial officials counted amongst opponents of the policy (Goerg, 1998; Gale, 1980). For instance, during his tenure as the principal colonial official in Gambia (1901–1911), Governor George Denton consistently opposed racial spatial segregation. The colonial official who voiced the loudest opposition to this policy was Governor William MacGregor, especially whilst governor of Lagos. MacGregor's opposition is particularly noteworthy because of his background as a medical doctor and a former colonial health official. Here, it is necessary to note that most members of the medical community were unified in arguing that segregation held the most promise as a strategy for protecting the health of colonial officials in Africa. On his part, MacGregor considered segregation foolhardy both as a health protection measure and a colonial governance strategy. His recommendation was for a comprehensive strategy to deal with malaria and other tropical diseases rather than segregation. Segregation, he argued, could only insignificantly reduce the incidence of disease in the European enclaves at best. Such a policy had no chance of combating malaria. This is because no more than nocturnal segregation was practical. Even then, as noted above, there were Africans who served Europeans in capacities that required them to spend nights or permanently live in European enclaves.

## Implications of colonial racial segregation

The socio-economic development implications of racially segregated spatial structures in Africa are discussed here in two segments. The first focuses on the colonial period while the second concentrates on the post-colonial era. Ultimately, the discussion demonstrates the counter-productive nature of racial spatial segregation as a health promotion/protection strategy.

### *The colonial era*

It is arguable that racial spatial segregation helped to boost the morale and comfort of Europeans in colonial Africa. However, any possible gains from segregation were neutralized or effaced by the problems it created or amplified. For instance, it has been suggested that segregation contributed enormously to destroying the social harmony that had always been present between Europeans and Africans. This was especially true in coastal towns. Such towns were racially integrated before racial spatial segregation became the official policy of colonial governments throughout the continent (Gale, 1980).

Segregation can also be criticized on moral and ethical grounds. On this score, the making of racially segregated spatial structures entailed using funds obtained from Africans through taxation or the sales of their natural resources to build and exorbitantly equip exclusive European enclaves. At the same time, such structures made it possible for non-European districts to be neglected or denied essential pieces of hygiene and sanitation infrastructure as well as other public services. In the Gold Coast (present-day Ghana), a colonial government report, *The Gold Coast Medical Report* for 1914 reported that African districts or towns saw their budgets for basic services significantly diminish as Europeans relocated to exclusive European enclaves (Gale, 1980).

Furthermore, segregation policies contributed enormously to the mistrust of Europeans by Africans. An important rationale for such policies as discussed above was that nocturnal segregation of the races was necessary as a prophylaxis against malaria for Europeans in colonial Africa. However, this rationale was rendered dubious by the actions of Europeans. In practice, authorities evicted higher-class Africans from European enclaves. However, as noted above, they were silent when it came to Africans who served Europeans in domestic and/or concubinary capacities. Such individuals continued living in exclusive European enclaves even after segregation had become official colonial policy. The cases of Bathurst, Lagos and Cape Coast are illustrative (Gale, 1980). In Bathurst and Lagos exclusive European enclaves continued to contain the servants and mistresses of Europeans after 1904 when racial residential segregation had become the official policy in Britain's tropical African colonies. In Cape Coast, African officials, but not prisoners and servants, were removed from the Castle as part of measures designed to actualize racial segregation policies in the colonies. These contradictory actions served to reinforce Africans' skepticism about the sincerity of the medical rationale for segregation policies. In fact, one African doctor is quoted as contending that European colonial authorities instituted spatial segregation not for medical reasons but as a means of asserting the European's contempt for, and authority and perceived superiority over, the African. In this vain, "the educated African is his [the European's] bug-bear; and ... that segregation is European snobbery crystallized" (Gale, 1980: 505).

A further negative consequence of racial segregation, especially on medical grounds is highlighted by the position of French colonial authorities in the same connection. By the twilight of the colonial era, the French had revised their stance on segregation. They were committed to winning the hearts and minds of the colonized. Therefore, they viewed racial segregation as antithetical to efforts to attain this objective. As part of their new philosophy on colonialism, they had promulgated new medical and health policies. These policies were designed to protect not only the health of the resident European population but also that of Africans. The French had come to see medical policy a viable form of political propaganda and a potent instrument for enlisting loyalty. Such loyalty was necessary as a prerequisite for cultivating the vast pool of healthy labourers and soldiers necessary for the colonial project's success. Failure to protect the health and welfare of Africans as segregationist policies were wont to do, would have contributed to the colonial project's failure.

*The post-colonial era*

Although it was supplanted by socio-economic class segregation in many parts subsequent to the demise of colonialism, racial residential segregation remains a fact of life in some parts of Africa. The cases of South Africa, Kenya, Zimbabwe (before Mugabe's controversial land reform initiatives of the 1990s), and Namibia are illustrative. Whatever the case, racial spatial segregation policies have far-reaching implications for contemporary development efforts throughout the continent. Foremost in this regard are the contributions of racially segregated spatial structures to: 1) socio-economic class-based cleavages, 2) transportation difficulties, and 3) health problems.

The contribution of colonial racially segregated spatial structures to socio-economic class-based cleavages in contemporary Africa can be understood by examining the redistribution of urban space subsequent to the demise of colonialism throughout the continent. The onset of independence witnessed the re-apportionment of urban space and concomitant facilities bequeathed to leaders of the emerging countries by colonial authorities. In this regard, the erstwhile exclusively European enclaves were assigned to senior government officials, while the areas that were occupied by elite members of the indigenous population were assigned to their mid-level colleagues. The formerly native districts were re-designated as the general residential district containing mostly low-income urban residents.

Thus, the distribution schema that was disproportionately skewed in favour of Europeans during the colonial era was re-tooled to advantage socio-economic elites following the demise of colonialism. Therefore, once colonialism ended in Africa, "racial segregation transformed into socio-economic and legal tenural residential segregation" (K'Akumu and Olima, 2007: 87). More noteworthy for the purpose of this discussion is the fact that the new spatial structure has resulted in severe population congestion and related problems such as the proliferation of slums in the general districts. For instance, as K'Akumu and Olima (2007: 87) have noted, an estimated 55 percent of the population of Nairobi lives in the general or low-income district, which constitutes only 5 percent of the city's residential area. Thus, contemporary urban development policies favour the residential areas of the elites while discriminating against the general or low-income areas of urban centres throughout Africa.

The re-apportionment of previously racially segregated urban space subsequent to the demise of colonialism ensured, among other things that the poor were heaped into the smallest and most undesirable areas. These areas soon degenerated into some of the worst slums found in Africa today. The slums typically contain immigrants from rural areas and other African countries. In Abidjan, Cote d'Ivoire's largest city, immigrants from neighbouring countries such as Burkina Faso, Mali, and Niger account for 60 percent of the population in the city's slums (UN-GRHS, 2009). As the population of such areas grow, their spatial isolation from the better off members of society increases. This is true even if the level of segregation remains constant (Massey and Denton, 1993). Physical isolation has implications for cultural and linguistic development (Ibid). Typically, slum residents tend to feel a sense of alienation that leads them to perceive the signs and messages of the dominant culture as hypocritical. Also worth noting is the fact that socio-economic class segregation, by definition, tends to concentrate poverty, crime and health problems in impoverished areas. Concomitant with this concentration is the absence of role models in low-income areas. Additionally, socio-economic class segregation contributes to excluding the poor from the political process. By being spatially isolated in impoverished districts, the poor usually have limited or no access to government institutions and are unable to establish alliances with influential societal groups.

Other negative implications of colonial racial spatial segregation policies surface in the area of urban transportation. Exclusive European residential districts and colonial government stations were, as part of efforts to physically separate Europeans from natives, located at considerable distances from non-European areas. As stated earlier, once colonialism ended, the indigenous leadership re-apportioned the districts in in erstwhile colonial cities. This resulted in physically separating the residential areas of upper- and mid-level government employees, and government offices from other areas in erstwhile colonial cities. Consequently, the residents of these cities, most of which serve as the capitals of African countries today, must travel long distances for government services. Also, workers in government or those serving in government residential areas tend to spend more time and/or money than otherwise necessary on work-related transportation.

## Conclusion

That urban space was segregated along racial lines in colonial Africa is incontestable. What remains uncertain is why colonial authorities, irrespective of background and ideological persuasion, decided in favour of racially segregated spatial structures. Most works on this subject are unified in attributing segregation policies to efforts to protect the health of Europeans in colonial Africa. This chapter has deviated from convention by contending that racism, informed by the race ideology of the nineteenth century, was at the root of these policies. It has been more than a century since the earliest and best-known of these policies were enacted. Almost half a century has elapsed since most African countries celebrated the demise of colonialism. However, the reverberations of racial segregation continue to be felt throughout the continent. Structures that used to be segregated along racial lines are today differentiated on the basis of socio-economic status. The problems associated with segregated spatial structures have only grown worse with the gap between the health and other conditions in upper-income districts and those in poor districts growing larger by the day. Thus, segregated spatial structures are not only of historic, but also of contemporary importance. Efforts to ameliorate health conditions in particular, and living conditions in general, in Africa cannot succeed without accounting for the implications of such structures.

# Chapter 5
# Public Health Implications of Modernist Planning

## Introduction

In his groundbreaking work on ancient African cities, Richard Hull (1976) draws attention to an important but oft-ignored fact about Africa. The fact is that complex and meticulously developed cities existed in Africa prior to the arrival of the first European on the continent. In particular, urban planning principles and practice were known in Africa before the European conquest. Thus, the term modernist planning is employed here to distinguish the planning that Europeans introduced, from the indigenous or traditional planning practiced by Africans. Particularly, the term modernist planning as employed here refers to the urban planning principles, methods and practice that developed subsequent to the industrial revolution in Western Europe (cf., UN-CHS, 2009).

A noteworthy aspect of modernist planning is the fact that soon after its development it was exported to other parts of the world. In Africa, this approach to urban planning was institutionalized and given concrete form by colonial authorities. Colonial authorities have been replaced in this capacity by agents of Westernization and modernization subsequent to the demise of colonialism throughout the continent. Like their colonial predecessors, agents of Westernization have sought to supplant indigenous spatial organization strategies and environmental standards with Western or so-called modern varieties. This chapter shows how supplanting indigenous African spatial and physical development strategies with Eurocentric varieties has contributed to the degradation, rather than the improvement, of health conditions on the continent. The chapter begins in the next section by highlighting some important characteristics of modernist spatial and physical planning with implications for public health.

## Characteristics of modernist urban planning

The structure of towns built on modernist planning principles in Africa differs markedly from that of the indigenous ones they supplanted. Indigenous African towns evolved from villages and hamlets. The growth of these towns was propelled mainly by internal factors such as religion, industry and commerce. Towns of great antiquity such as Kano, Nigeria and Great Zimbabwe in present day Zimbabwe developed as religious centres. Kumasi, which attained the zenith of its popularity as the capital of the Asante confederacy in present-day Ghana, blossomed as a great centre of commerce. Thus, the growth of indigenous African cities was mainly a function of internal as opposed to external forces. More noteworthy for the purpose of the discussion in this chapter is the fact that indigenous African cities developed in a compact and sustainable fashion.

In contrast, the cities that were established by Europeans, especially during the colonial era, developed in response to external forces. In fact, the cities served a crucial function as locales for colonial government administration and the transitory handling of natural resources slated for onward transmission to colonial master nations. Thus, the cities that were created by Europeans served an important role in the European colonial project in Africa. For this and cognate reasons, the cities were developed on modernist planning principles. Distinct features of these cities include the fact that their development is strictly regulated by or incorporate:

- The zoning ordinance;
- Western laws designed to compartmentalize land use activities;
- Eurocentric building codes and other formal building regulatory instruments;
- Eurocentric housing standards; and
- Eurocentric land tenure systems.

As shown in Table 5.1, and elaborated below, each of these features of modernist planning has far-reaching implications for public health in Africa.

**Table 5.1 Public health implications of modernist planning**

| Modernist planning feature | Intended purpose | Unintended health implications |
|---|---|---|
| zoning | Separate incompatible land use activities in order to promote and protect public health | In practice, zoning serves to worsen the health conditions of the poor by confining them to areas that:<br>• are by nature unhealthy;<br>• have been rendered unhealthy because they are not provided with basic services;<br>• double as waste dump sites; and/or<br>• serve as the site for locally undesired land use activities. |
| Compartmentalization of land use activities | Promote efficient and effective use of land | Results in elongating distances between activity points. The distances are usually too long for walking, thereby encouraging dependence on motorized means of transportation. Thus, opportunities for passive exercising are eliminated. |
| Building standards and codes | Ensure the safety of occupants and users of buildings; promote general public health | Policies falling under this rubric contribute to the problem of homelessness at worst, and housing shortage at best. Both problems in turn contribute to poor health. |
| Housing standards | Promote public health | The acceptable number of persons that occupy any given space or room is a function of culture. Eurocentric prescriptions in this regard tend to clash with African culture. Hence, to the extent that health, from a holistic perspective, encompasses culture, we contend that the Eurocentric housing standards do not promote health in Africa. |
| Use of Eurocentric land tenure system | Ensure security of tenure; promote economic development by facilitating the transfer of land | Contributes to the landlessness problem among the poor; Leads the poor to resort to living on precarious and unhealthy locales. |

*Zoning and its impact on public health*

Zoning originated in Western Europe in the 1800s. At the time, its main objective was to ensure a safe distance between noxious land use activities on the one hand, and residential and cognate uses on the other. Since then, it has been adopted as the primary instrument for governing the timing and location of land use activities in developed and developing countries alike. In its simplest form, zoning is employed to divide land within any defined municipality, local government area, city or town, into broad categories such as residential, commercial, and industrial. These are further divided into single family and multiple family (residential); and light and heavy industrial uses. In essence, zoning ordinances specify activities that can, or cannot, take place in any given location.

The avowed aim of zoning is to protect the health, lives, and safety of land users. In theory, therefore, zoning strives to protect the health and safety of everyone within any given municipality. However, as demonstrated in this book, this is hardly the case in practice. In practice, zoning strives to protect the health, safety, and economic and related interests of the preferred societal groups. This does not nullify the fact that urban planning is tied to public health through zoning. In fact, as Schilling and Linton (2005: 96) have noted,

> zoning and public health laws evolved from the same legal ancestors—the common law of public nuisance and the expansion of state police powers, both premised on protection of the public's health.

Yet, even the most ardent proponents of zoning as an instrument for protecting public health are quick to make the following concession. Since it was initially proposed as an instrument for the protection of the public's health, zoning has evolved to take on responsibilities that cannot be logically connected to health. In this regard, Schilling and Linton (2005) invoke the 1926 landmark decision of the U.S. Supreme Court in the *Ambler Realty v. Village of Euclid* case as evidence that zoning in the United is more about the protection of property rights than about the protection of public health. To be sure, the *Ambler Realty v. Village of Euclid* case does, albeit nominally, recognize the health basis of zoning.

The court decisions that have been rendered with respect to zoning in the United States since 1926 have been largely oblivious to the public health implications of zoning. More recently, zoning in the U.S. has been criticized for causing urban sprawl, the loss of wilderness and farmland, racial and socio-economic segregation, and the channelling of resources to privileged neighbourhoods at the expense of impoverished ones (Hall, 2007).

As an instrument of land use control, zoning was introduced in Africa by colonial authorities. It was essentially part of the broader colonial project to supplant indigenous models of spatial organization with European varieties. The variable promotion and protection of public health based on their geographic location, which was tied to other human characteristics, particularly 'race,' is a colonial legacy in Africa. Colonial urban planning principles and practice dictated the separation of European enclaves from the native areas not only by physical distance. Rather, a distinguishing mark between the two areas was the extent to which each was equipped with utility services, physical and social amenities. In this regard, the spacious facilities of the European enclaves were developed to the physical and environmental standards in vogue in Europe at the time. Thus, these facilities were equipped with electricity, pipe borne water and well aligned, named and sign-posted streets. In addition, houses and other buildings in these enclaves were numbered. In contrast, none of these amenities was provided in the so-called native areas.

Zoning was employed in Africa mainly as an instrument to compartmentalize the built environment along racial lines. For instance, in eastern and southern Africa, colonial authorities used zoning to compartmentalize residential areas into three main districts, comprising the European enclave, the 'coloured' district and the 'native' district. The disease theory of the time suggested that high altitudes helped to promote good health. Consequently, colonial authorities selected high altitudes as the location of choice for European enclaves. Conversely, they designated low-lying areas as the residential districts of Africans. Therefore, the health benefits believed to be associated with high altitudes were never extended to members of the native population. This is because, based on the racist ideology of the time, Africans were dispensable.

Subsequent to the demise of colonialism, the residential districts were re-named and re-assigned to different classes within the emerging nations. In this regard, the European enclaves, which were zoned to have the lowest density, were inherited by elite members of the indigenous society. The 'coloured' districts, which were zoned as medium density, were assigned to middle-income members of the society. The 'native' districts, zoned as high density, were assigned to the poor. Authorities in colonial Zimbabwe also operated a three-tier racial classification system, which was used to determine the differential manner in which different groups would benefit from health and sanitation infrastructure and services. As Rakodi (1986) noted, the system placed Europeans at the top of the pyramidal racial classification structure, while Asians occupied the middle rung and Blacks were at the bottom.

To illustrate the differential distribution of health and sanitation infrastructure and services, Rakodi draws on the case of Ndola, one of the local municipalities. Here, the White residential areas were generously equipped with sanitation and cognate amenities, including in-door plumbing, large residential units, gardens, and well-maintained lighted streets. In contrast, the African neighbourhood had very little, if any sanitary facilities. In the mid-1930s this neighbourhood had a population of 4000 cramped into as few as 1,700 mud huts and access to only 50 pit latrines, with hardly any other sanitary facility (Rakodi, 1986: 198).

Thus, apart from physically confining people to pre-determined areas based on some arbitrary characteristic, zoning has also proved effective in influencing the (re)distribution of social and economic resources. As shown in the case of colonial Zimbabwe, health and related public infrastructure and services, such as water and sanitation facilities, were provided in European enclaves but not in the so-called native districts.

At the end of the colonial era, and the concomitant departure of Europeans, the indigenous leadership assumed control of the colonial government offices, and re-assigned the erstwhile European enclaves to members of the upper echelons of what at the time was an emerging independent government bureaucracy. At the same time, they designated the erstwhile native areas as the residential district of low-income members of the society. While the upper-income areas continued to benefit from some degree of upkeep and maintenance, particularly in terms of utility provisioning and planning code enforcement, the low-income areas were virtually neglected. With the passage of time, the low-income areas have grown to unprecedented levels as deteriorating conditions in rural areas increasingly result in mass rural-to-urban migration. With the demise of colonialism, racial spatial segregation has effectively been transformed into socio-economic spatial segregation.

Thus, the pattern of resource distribution established during the colonial era has since been maintained by indigenous authorities. Consequently, the upper-income and the middle-income districts have access to water, health and related services while the poor ones do not. To compound this situation, the poor districts are usually the smallest in terms of land mass but the largest in terms of population size. The case of Nairobi, Kenya, exemplifies this situation (see Box 5.1). Here, as much as 60 per cent of the city's population live in slums that take up no more than 5 per cent of the city's land area (Warah, 2010). The health problems resulting from the exceedingly high density, compounded by the absence of basic services in the slums are obvious. A quick glance at one of Nairobi's slums, Kibera, reputed as the second largest slum in Africa, and one of the largest in world, is revelatory in this regard. The United Nations Centre for Human Settlements (UN-Habitat) reported that Kibera, with a population of 700,000, had a density of 2000 persons per hectare in 2003 (UN-Habitat, 2003). The slum is characterized as "heavily polluted by human refuse, garbage, soot, dust, and other wastes" (Warah, 2010). In addition, it is contaminated with human and animal feces, occasioned by open sewage and the lack of toilet facilities. The spatial injustice engendered by such inequitable distribution of basic infrastructure and services, is therefore, a colonial legacy. In particular, it is a product of modernist planning initiatives under the rubric of zoning. Therefore, despite its avowed aim of ensuring the health, safety, and welfare of the general public, zoning in Africa has in reality, been exclusionary as it differentially promotes and protects the health of different segments of the public.

Indigenous leaders throughout Africa have religiously adhered to the spirit of the spatial organization blueprint bequeathed to them by their colonial predecessors. The zoning ordinance constitutes a major component of this blueprint. At the same time, it is a prominent feature of the master plans that have been drawn up mainly by Western planning consultants for towns throughout the continent. Within the framework of a typical modernist master plan, a town is divided up into four major types of districts, namely residential, business, industrial and public (Njoh, 2003: 154). The residential district is further divided into three distinct areas, including high-density, medium density, and low density, roughly corresponding with the locales for low-income, medium-income and high-income housing facilities respectively.

The noted inequalities and especially the increasingly worsening economic condition of residents of the densely packed districts do not bode well for their health. As Wang'ombe (1995) once noted, the public health situation in such districts is seriously threatened not because the residents fall sick more often than their counterparts in other areas but because of a number of related factors. Prominent in this regard are the diseases associated with poverty and the unavailability of, and inaccessibility to, basic health services. Here, it is important to note that the high levels of poverty that constitute a defining characteristic of African countries are concentrated in the low-income or poor districts of urban areas.

**Box 5.1 Modernist planning and the making of slums in Africa:**
**The case of Kibera, Nairobi**

Kibera is reputed as Kenya's largest slum and the second largest in Africa. Credit for the slum's creation is due to British colonial authorities. However, Kenya's indigenous authorities deserve credit for enacting the land, spatial development and cognate policies that fueled its growth and development. British colonial authorities established Kibera as a locale to re-settle Nubian soldiers, who had served in the British military during the First World War. Colonial authorities saw no need to enforce town planning rules in the settlement, which consequently developed on an informal basis. When Kenya gained political independence in 1963, the indigenous leadership, allured by the modernization ideology, moved with unparalleled gusto to outlaw informal settlements. This move resulted in making Kibera an 'illegal settlement' wherein all residents were in violation of one or more of a number of town planning statutes. Consequently, instead of working to improve living conditions, the post-colonial state took every step possible to discourage living in the settlement. Among the most egregious of these steps was refusal to neither make more land available for possible expansion nor provide residents with basic sanitation and other services. Despite these and other tactics on the part of the government, the population of the settlement continued to grow by leaps and bounds. Today, Kibera stands out as one of the most densely populated, unhygienic, insalubrious and unhealthy slums in the world.

*Source*: Adapted from Wikipedia.com.

The proportion of the total population living below the extreme poverty line in urban areas in Africa rose from 66 million in 1993 to 99 million in 2002 (UN-CHS, 2009: 37). More noteworthy especially because of its public health implications is the fact that Africa boasts not only the highest incidence of urban poverty (over 40 per cent per cent) but also the largest proportion of urban residents (62 per cent) living in slums (UN-CHS, 2009: 37). Leading on this score are countries such as Angola, Chad, the Central African Republic, Ethiopia, Guinea Bissau, Madagascar, Niger, Sierra Leone, Sudan and Uganda. The frequent outbreaks of epidemics that have wreaked havoc in some of these countries in the recent past have originated in slums. In fact, slums such as those in Nairobi, Kenya are notorious for annual cholera outbreaks during the rainy season (Wang'ombe, 1995).

Although a universal phenomenon, the inequitable distribution of public infrastructure and access to important services, including healthcare, is exaggerated in Africa. Here, to be poor and living in the poor districts of urban centres is not to have access to health services. For instance, it has been noted that women and children in such districts have little or no access to maternal and child health services (Wang'ombe, 1995). In addition, such districts experience more than their own share of outbreaks of epidemics of immunizable diseases and diseases of nutritional deficiency as well as AIDS and other sexually transmissible diseases (Ibid).

Such areas are also more deficient in terms of vital communication infrastructure and services such as telephones, streets wide enough for motorized vehicular traffic, electricity, and water. The implications of such deficiencies for public health are far-reaching. For example, residents of poor districts or slums are not able to summon the assistance of medical emergency units or ambulances when they are suddenly taken ill. Similarly, they cannot call on the fire department in the event of a fire. For one thing, these residents have no telephones through which they can call on such services. For another thing, there are no streets wide enough for emergency or any other vehicle for that matter in these districts. The absence of accessible roads in poor districts and slums also tends to encourage criminal activities as they are typically inaccessible to elements of law and order. Thus, apart from issues of health, these districts also face safety and security problems.

The problem of inequitable distribution of resources also presents itself in Africa in terms of the geographic location of the privileged and underprivileged. Again, this problem is rooted in colonial modernist planning schemes, and maintained by contemporary zoning legislation. It is articulated in the differential location of upper- and middle-income districts on the best sites and the poor districts in precarious locales.

One specific example serves to illuminate this phenomenon. French colonial authorities in the People's Republic of Congo located two neighbourhoods designed to serve as the exclusive district of members of the native population in Brazzaville in a swampy area known as Poto Poto. In contrast, these authorities located the exclusive European enclave on the most precinct and elevated area in the city. It is for this reason that swampy Poto Poto remains the locale of present-day Brazzaville's worst slum. Brazzaville is not unique in this regard. The Kibera slum in Nairobi, Kenya mentioned earlier, sits on a precarious piece of land on the shores of the Nairobi River, and close to the Nairobi Dam. Makoko, a well-known slum in Lagos Nigeria, is located literally on water in one of the city's most precarious creeks. Similarly, Quartier Nylon and Quartier Bepanda in Douala, Cameroon are located in areas notorious for flooding and severe drainage problems. In general, such districts, because of their location, constitute dumpsites or collection points for rainwater, effluent and other wastes from residential quarters and industrial plants. The stagnant water and overgrown shrubbery and bushes at such points in turn serve as breeding sites for disease vectors such as mosquitoes and rodents.

The ability of modernist planning instruments such as zoning to confine different socio-economic groups to different geographic regions or districts within a city, town or village makes it possible for policy makers to neglect districts occupied by the less powerful and already disenfranchised groups. Although critics have done well to draw attention to the negative implications of zoning, they appear consistently oblivious to the instrument's impact on public health. One such impact is pollution, which results from the excessive dependence on motorized forms of transportation occasioned by elongated distances between activity points.

## Compartmentalization of land use activities

At one level, the compartmentalization of land use activities in urban planning is designed to achieve some of the same goals as zoning. However, at another level, compartmentalization has different objectives that can best be understood in the context of its origins. Compartmentalization is a product of the Enlightenment period. In fact, some have characterized modernist planning in general as a product of the Enlightenment belief that the rational transformation of urban space would lead to the social betterment of urban residents (see e.g., Papayanis, 2004). Seen from this perspective, land use compartmentalization resulted not only from the need to protect the health and safety of urban residents—as did zoning. Rather, it also resulted from the need to promote order and functionality in urban space according to Enlightenment principles.

In Africa, colonial urban planners defined spatial order to include among other things, spatially segregating the races. In this regard, it is worth noting that the choice of high altitudes as the location of choice for European enclaves had only little to do with health. Rather, it had everything to do with the need to control and dominate Africans as well as maintain order in urban areas. Thus, the differential location of European enclaves vis-à-vis the 'native' districts was designed to blatantly accentuate the socio-psychological difference between the 'ruler' and the 'ruled.' With the demise of colonialism, as stated earlier, the bureaucratic and military elites of the indigenous societies took over the residential units in the formerly exclusive European enclaves. Concomitant with this was the inheritance of the colonial government offices by the post-colonial government authorities. In addition, spatial order also meant physically separating residential districts from office parks. For instance, the German colonial government plan for Douala,

Cameroon, included a one-kilometer-wide green belt that separated the European enclave and colonial government office park in Bonanjo from the native areas in Deido and New Akwa, as well as the non-indigenous African area in New Bell (Njoh, 2006; Schler, 2003).

The compartmentalized spatial structures did not go away with colonialism. Rather, they constitute the nucleus around which contemporary modern cities throughout Africa have developed. One upshot of the resultant spatial structures is that they effectively contribute to thwarting ongoing health and safety promotion efforts in African cities. It is paradoxical that structures that had as their avowed aim, the protection of public health, now serve to obfuscate health promotion initiatives. To be sure, this paradox is not unique to Africa. Rather, as noted in a study commissioned by the US-based Transportation Research Board (TRB, 2005), the paradox is also well-known in the United States and other parts of North America. In the US, for example, urban reformers recommended low density development and the segregation of land use activities with a view to reducing the spread of diseases associated with overcrowded human settlements. Today, these recommendations effectively thwart efforts designed to promote healthy lifestyles that depend on non-motorized means of locomotion. In this case, some have pondered whether the dispersed spatial structures, hence largely automobile-dependent development patterns that were created by land use compartmentalization are at the root of the physically inactive or sedentary lifestyles of most Americans (TRB, 2005: vii).

Studies such as the afore-cited that seek to interrogate the implications of features of the built environment for public health have largely focused on developed regions. These studies have seldom focused on developing regions such as Africa. Yet, because the spatial structure of the built environment in Africa was designed to accomplish multiple, and sometimes, conflicting goals, its implications for public health are likely to be a lot more far-reaching.

Clearly, the dispersal of land use activities over vast geographic space has health implications that may either be positive or negative. On the positive side, the dispersal of land use activities occasioned by land use compartmentalization can compel people to indulge in passive physical activities as they get from one activity point to another within the built environment. Evidence abounds to the effect that physical activity, including walking, contributes to preventing the development of numerous chronic diseases, improves psychological well-being, and reduces the risk of premature mortality (TRB, 2005). However, it is important to note that the point at which spatial dispersion can turn from benefiting to hurting efforts to improve public health is unclear. It would appear that only initiatives to disperse land use activities undertaken with the specific aim of promoting passive exercising have the greatest chance of succeeding in this regard.

As noted above, the compartmentalization of land use activities in Africa was designed to accomplish goals far-removed from promoting passive exercising. Today, inhabitants of the erstwhile colonial cities are compelled to spend their meagre resources on motorized means of transportation. This is because the distances separating different activity points in these cities are too vast to negotiate on foot. For instance, in the city of Kumba, Cameroon, the distance separating the Government Station from Kumba Town is at least 8 kilometers (Njoh, 1997: 136). In Bamenda, another Cameroonian city, the hilltop-located Government Station is linked to Bamenda Town, located at the foot of the hill, by a meandering highway etched into a steep rocky hill. When British colonial authorities developed one of Africa's most famous (or infamous, depending on one's ideological orientation) hill stations in Freetown, Sierra Leone in 1904, it was connected to the main town by a narrow gauge, custom-built 'mountain railway' (Njoh, 1999; Frenkel and Western, 1988). In the afore-described and similar cases throughout Africa, the resultant spatial structure creates unnecessary reliance on motorized means of transportation. The public health consequences of this phenomenon are obvious and include, but are not limited to:

- possible injuries and fatalities (to drivers, passengers, and pedestrians) that are directly related to motorized transportation services, and air pollution;
- air pollution resulting from the exhaust fumes of motorized vehicles;
- decreased physical activity, as people become dependent on motorized means of locomotion; and
- poverty, as scarce individual financial resources are spent on defraying the cost of transportation instead of more important basic needs such as food and shelter.

The World Health Organization has identified traffic injuries as a leading cause of death worldwide (WHO and World Bank, 2004). In 2002, Africa had a traffic accident fatality rate in excess of 28 per 100,000, which was the highest of all low-income regions in the world (WHO and World Bank, 2004: 34). Most of these accidents occur on urban streets as opposed to highways. For instance, recent statistics from Ethiopia reveal that as much as 68 per cent of all traffic accidents in that country occur in urban areas as compared to only 19 per cent that occur in rural areas (Abiye, 2009).

The excessive dependence on motorized transportation occasioned by elongated distances between points of activities in geographic space causes other health problems. For example, the long periods spent on buses, taxi cabs or other passenger vehicles can be stressful. In addition, delays necessitated by unnecessarily long distances between activity points takes away from time that could have been used for relaxation or recreation purposes.

Despite the vast distances separating activity points in African countries, a good many have no choice but to go about on foot. It is true that walking is recommended for healthy living. However, trekking is often not only tiring but actually dangerous in these countries. The fact that pedestrians are widely believed to be the most vulnerable road users in African cities lends credence to this assertion. In fact, as much as 65 per cent of road traffic-related injuries and deaths in Mozambique, for instance, involve pedestrians (Washington Post, 2007). Also worth noting is the fact that people trekking for long distances through non-activity areas risk being mugged or attacked. In fact, in Kumba, Cameroon, such crimes are known to frequently victimize informal sector women making the long trek from the Government Station to Kumba Town (Njoh, 1995).

### Modernist building standards and codes

The building codes and standards that constitute an important element of modernist urban planning in Africa were inherited from the continent's colonial past. The motivation for introducing the codes and standards in Africa can be explained at four different but overlapping levels. First, the European colonial authorities who introduced the codes and standards in Africa originated in a region, namely Europe, with vast experience in dealing with the negative externalities of industrialization and concomitant urbanization. Developments in Europe, especially during the eighteenth century, had prompted social reformers such as Edwin Chadwick and Friedrich Engels to issue some of the most authoritative statements on the negative consequences of industrialization and the urbanization it engendered. Chadwick's 1842 Report on *The Sanitary Conditions of the Labouring Population of Great Britain*, and Engel's 1844 classic on *The Conditions of the Working Classes in 1844* are especially noteworthy in this connection. They linked living conditions and amenities to disease. At the same time, these reformers drew attention to the need for policy makers to formulate laws and policies capable of mitigating especially the health problems associated with the twin phenomena of industrialization and urbanization. Among the many upshots of these are the enactment of Britain's first Public Health Act in 1848 and the building codes that were promulgated throughout Western Europe and other parts of the Western world at the time. With the advent of the European colonial era, authorities found it convenient to simply transplant to Africa the codes that were already in force in the West.

A second explanation is rooted in the race ideology that was in vogue at the time. Thus, Europeans deemed it necessary to simply supplant the 'inferior African traditional building standards' with the 'superior European variety.' The third explanation has to do with an important objective of European colonialism, namely to promote economic development in Europe. In this regard, the codes, especially those of the prescriptive variant, sought to promote the sale of building materials, techniques and skills originating in Europe. Lastly, the laws can be viewed as a product of the desire on the part of agents of Western civilization to promote pseudo-Western environmental standards in Africa. Essentially, these agents have bought into Western propaganda campaigns designed to herald Eurocentric standards as superior and universal. In other words, there is a burning desire on the part of indigenous authorities throughout Africa to modernize their countries. This desire is at the root of contemporary policies that seek to promote building materials imported from the West, while branding the local or traditional equivalents as 'primitive,' 'substandard,' and unhealthy. Within the framework of the race ideology that was in vogue in the eighteenth century, proper hygiene and sanitation in human settlements could be achieved only through the adoption of Euro-centric physical structures and standards. Consequently, as noted earlier, physical structures, particularly housing units built of traditional and improvised materials were considered unhealthy and unfit for habitation.

Agents of modernization have always viewed every phenomenon with Eurocentric roots as universal. Yet, nothing could be further from the truth, especially with regards to building construction and environmental standards. Human beings, regardless of their location, have always found a way to meet the critical need of shelter. Prior to the move towards modernization, Africans addressed this need with locally available materials, which were both in ample supply and affordable. However, efforts to 'modernize' the continent have resulted in a proclivity towards imported materials. As far back as the 1970s, the doyen of affordable housing in developing countries, J.F.C. Turner (1972), had pondered how authorities in these countries would afford the Eurocentric standards that they seek to promote given their scant resource base.

Building standards are typically of two varieties, namely the prescriptive-oriented and the performance-based. Both types have as their avowed aim, the promotion and protection of the health, safety and welfare of building occupants as well as the public at large. Performance-oriented codes typically recommend the (performance) objective to be accomplished and allow broad leeway to the building designer to select the materials and methods necessary to attain the desired results. For example, the performance code for walls may stipulate the standards that walls must meet, such as load bearing capacity, sound, heat, and fire resistance. It may also require that the walls be capable of counteracting excessive deflection and withstanding possible vibration. In contrast, a specification-oriented code stipulates, with precision, the materials and construction techniques that must be employed for various components of the building. For example, a specification for wood-frame construction typically includes precise dimensions for the size and spacing of wood studs, allowable spans for floor joists, and the number of nails required for connecting wood members. Authorities working under a specification-oriented regime, on the one hand, usually stipulate that building construction be undertaken only by formally trained technicians, working under the auspices of formally registered building contractors. On the other hand, those adhering to the principles of performance-oriented standards are likely to simply state the performance standards that the completed building or components thereof must meet. Consequently, the owner and builder are at liberty to select the materials necessary to meet those standards.

*Public health implications of modernist building standards*

Two consequences of prescriptive standards that favour imported building materials as opposed to materials of the domestic genre have direct public health implications. One of the consequences is housing shortage, and the other is poverty (Njoh, 1999). The problem of housing shortage in Africa is, at least in part, a direct result of efforts to duplicate Western environmental standards on the continent. Paradoxically, these efforts are usually masqueraded as initiatives to promote public health. Prominent in this regard are the schemes that are typically designed to eradicate slum and squatter settlements. Here, as was the case in Western Europe and North America in the 1800s and early-1900s, authorities in Africa have moved to clear housing units that do not meet the modernist planner's definition of 'standard housing.' Note that an overwhelming majority of housing in Africa fails the litmus test for 'standard housing' and therefore, qualifies as 'slum housing.' The UN-Habitat (2007) defines slum housing as non-durable housing, where more than three persons share the same room, and do not have easy access to adequate sanitation facilities such as a private or public toilet that is shared by few people. In the words of the UN-Habitat itself, a slum dwelling is one that lacks one or more of the following (Ibid, para. 1):

- Durable housing of a permanent nature that protects against extreme climate conditions;
- Sufficient living space which means not more than three people sharing the same room;
- Easy access to safe water in sufficient amounts at an affordable price;
- Access to adequate sanitation in the form of a private or public toilet shared by a reasonable number of people; and
- Security of tenure that prevents forced evictions.

Throughout Africa, particularly in the 1970s and 1980s, governments were busy demolishing so-called slums on the pretext that they were unsanitary, unhealthy and aesthetically unappealing features of the urban landscape. When the military government took over power in Nigeria in 1983, for instance, it wasted no time to adopt policies that it contended were designed to modernize, and improve the health of, Nigerian cities. One analyst has remarked that the Nigerian military authorities' policies "were nothing short of an impersonation of America's urban renewal projects of the 1960s" (Njoh, 1999: 161).

In the 1970s, the political and bureaucratic leaders in Senegal insisted on instituting unrealistic high minimum building and environmental standards in the country is capital city of Dakar. Accordingly, they ordered the mass clearance of so-called slum settlements as a means of modernizing the capital city's physical structure (Njoh, 1999; Simon, 1992). In Tanzania, this practice was discontinued in 1969 but re-introduced in the 1980s as the country strived to rid its urban centres of 'unhealthy,' 'undesirable' and 'shameful' features, and above all, give them a 'modern look' (Njoh, 1999; Lugalla, 1995). Although advertised as projects designed to promote public health, Tanzania's slum clearance schemes, as Lugalla (1995: 65) noted, had modernization objectives. The fact that so-called slums were/are usually replaced by ultra-modern office complexes, factories and hotels, bolsters Lugalla's assertion.

The problem is that, while authorities in Africa have been hasty to destroy, they have made hardly any effort to replace, the so-called slums. This invariably causes a significant housing shortage as occupants of the destroyed units are rendered homeless and/or forced to share housing with friends and relatives. Housing shortage or quantitative deficiencies in the housing market, in turn, lead to overcrowding as the population strives to make do with the limited number of housing units available. There is a wide range of definitions of overcrowding. One reason for this is that the concept of overcrowding has cultural connotations. In Western societies, the standard is to have one person per bedroom or two persons per bedroom if they are related by marriage or romance. However, in most African and other non-Western cultures, one person occupying a whole bedroom by him/herself would be considered lonely and/or selfish. In such societies, it is common for whole families to share sleeping quarters.

*Overcrowding and health*

Common sense suggests that, regardless of cultural variations, there is a limit to how many persons can healthily occupy any specific enclosed space at any given time. To the extent that this is true, overcrowding can be defined as follows (cf., US-HUD, 2007):

- in terms of the number of persons per bedroom in a dwelling unit;
- the number of persons per unit; the ratio of persons to floor space in square meters; and
- the person-to-size ratio adjusted for household composition, structure type, location, or lot size.

However, making a direct connection between overcrowding and health can prove to be a daunting task. A few studies, focusing exclusively on developed countries have attempted to make this connection. However, the findings of these studies essentially fail the face validity test. One such study sought to link mortality rates to aspects of housing, including overcrowding in England and Wales (see Fox and Goldblatt, 1982). The study revealed that female occupants of local authority rented housing who lived in units with 1.5 or more persons per room had a significantly higher mortality rate than those in units with less than 0.75 persons per room (Fox and Goldblatt, 1982). Studies of this kind constitute the basis for the view of one person per room, or two romantically related persons per room as ideal. Yet, there are serious difficulties inherent in isolating the impacts on health occasioned by overcrowding from those resulting from other housing deprivation-related variables (ODPM, 2004). While intuition or common sense may suggest a link between overcrowding and health, it is certainly not clear if an empirical link exists between these two variables. To be sure, some of the causal links that have been made especially between overcrowding and infectious diseases are intuitively appealing. For instance, overcrowding has been linked to tuberculosis and respiratory ailments (ODPM, 2004).

Also, because overcrowding implies congestion within any specific space, it is reasonable to suspect that there are physical health risks associated with overcrowding. Two studies, one conducted in England, and the other in the United States, provide some empirical evidence in this regard. The former, which was conducted by Alwash and McCarthy (1988) examined 400 child accident victims in a West London hospital and found that most domestic accident victims were likely to come from homes with more than 1.5 persons per room. The latter study was by Anderson and colleagues (1998). It revealed that child domestic accident victims with non-Hispanic background were likely to come from neighbourhoods with household overcrowding rates in excess of more than one person per room. This evidence suggests that overcrowding and health are somewhat related. However, the lack of empirical evidence from Africa, or other developing regions, on this and related questions leaves one to doubt if these findings have any universal implications. Yet, it is conceivable that regardless of culture, geographic location and other variables, the tighter the space, the higher the likelihood of domestic accidents. It is reasonable to expect the incidence of such accidents to be greater in impoverished locales where lighting is likely to be poor at best and non-existent at worst.

*Poverty and health*

The link between social factors and public health can be easily appreciated by simply imagining the cost implications and affordability issues inherent in coming by the basic amenities of life, including shelter, food, clean water, and so on. Within the context of this chapter, it is argued that high required minimum housing standards, and prescriptive-oriented building codes that encourage the use of Eurocentric building materials, make housing prohibitively costly for the poor. Consequently, poor and low-income families are compelled to spend a disproportionate proportion of their income on housing, thereby foregoing other basic necessities. Alternatively, such requirements may result in the poor consuming less than the desired quantity and quality of housing. Both options have health implications.

A few works have already identified poverty as a leading cause of health problems in Africa (see e.g., Mathee et al., 2009; Cooke, 2009). A recent report on *Public Health in Africa* by the Center for Strategic and International Studies pinpoints poverty and underdevelopment in general as leading causes of Africa's public health problematic (Cooke, 2009). In this regard, the report states as follows (Ibid, p. 1):

> The continent's immense disease burden and frail health systems are embedded in a broader context of poverty, underdevelopment, conflict and weak ill-managed government institutions.

To the extent that the high required minimum housing standards prescribed under the banner of modernist urban planning contributes to poverty, modernist planning can be said to play a role in creating a health-poverty vicious circle. In this connection, health and poverty are said to be related in a reciprocal or mutual fashion. In other words, poverty does not simply result from spending meagre resources on health services. Rather, ill-health itself tends to be at the root of poverty. This is because ill-health prevents people from effectively contributing to the economic production process. Thus, on the one hand, ill-health resulting from overcrowded or other forms of unhealthy housing contributes to poverty. On the other hand, poverty resulting from the fact that modernist building codes force people to spend a disproportionate amount of their incomes on housing.

## Conclusion

This chapter incriminates efforts to promote modernist planning as a source of some of the major public health problems that are commonplace within the built environment in Africa. In particular, it has argued that the minimum required environmental and building standards that authorities insist on enforcing tend to make housing less affordable. In essence therefore, such standards can be seen as a leading cause of the problem of homelessness, the growth and proliferation of slum settlements, as well as increasing levels of poverty. All of these problems have health implications. Here, policy makers in African countries are implored to eschew the temptation of insisting on environmental standards borrowed from Western countries. In this regard, these authorities must seek to promote locally available materials, which are definitely less expensive than the imported equivalents. To do so is to make housing more affordable, thereby dealing with the twin problem of qualitative and quantitative deficiencies in the housing market. More importantly, these authorities must avoid employing Eurocentric concepts of overcrowding. For one thing, the few studies on this subject, which by the way, have been conducted exclusively in Western countries are inconclusive. For another thing, the notion of health as defined by the World Health Organization (WHO), the authority charged with the responsibility for promoting global health within the United Nations is multi-dimensional and holistic. According to WHO (e.g., 2008) health comprises three dimensions of well-being, including physical, mental, and social. From the perspective of the WHO, therefore, health also depends on such aspects of life as one's social environment, and psychological state. Therefore, it would be foolhardy to abandon aspects of African indigenous culture that promote social cohesion and conversely frowns on any attempts to promote individualism, especially in the use of scarce resources such as domestic space.

# Chapter 6
# Hygiene and Sanitation Conditions in West and Central Africa

## Introduction

The undersupply of sanitation infrastructure constitutes a viable explanation for the fact that as many as 1.1 billion people in the developing world defecate in the open (WHO/UNICEF, 2010). In comparison to the situation a decade or so ago, this figure reflects a decline. The World Health Organization (WHO) and the United Nations Children's Fund (UNICEF) Joint Monitoring Programme for Water and Sanitation (JMP) (WHO/UNICEF, 2010: 22) noted a decline from 25 to 17 per cent in the global population that practices open defecation between 1990 and 2008.

The problem of inadequate sanitation infrastructure and services continues to be one of Africa's most nagging quandaries. Sanitation coverage on the continent remains the lowest of all major regions. Available statistics suggest that the situation is deteriorating (see e.g., WHO/UNICEF, 2008). Even in areas of apparent progress, the picture leaves much to be desired. Consider the following statistics as reported by the WHO/UNICEF (see WHO/UNICEF, 2010: 22). The continent enjoyed a decline in the proportion of people practicing open defecation between 1990 and 2006. However, the absolute number indulging in this practice actually increased from 188 million to 224 million during the same period.

Yet, it would be misleading to generalize the problem of poor sanitation to the entire continent. To be sure, the problem varies in both qualitative and quantitative terms from one region to another. It also differs markedly from one country to another. This chapter is dedicated to highlighting sanitation conditions in the West and Central Africa region. The importance of appreciating sanitation conditions in their regional contexts cannot be overstated. Such an appreciation can serve as a logical starting point for any meaningful efforts to ameliorate the conditions. Is the problem a function of history, geography, culture, politics, or economics? Also, an appreciation of the conditions in their regional or geographic contexts can lead to a more judicious allocation of resources. This is particularly important when such allocation involves agents of international development. The spending decisions of these entities in developing regions are often based on secondary information as opposed to information they collect themselves. A conversation on international activities in the water and sanitation domain in Africa is especially timely. This is especially because these activities have been intensified in the recent past. One factor accounting for the intensification of these activities is an increased awareness of the correlation between insalubrious conditions and poor health. Another factor is the need to meet water-and-sanitation-related targets of the Millennium Development Goals (MDGs). A perusal of the Millennium Development Goals reveals that none of the goals can been attained without increased access to improved water and sanitation. Yet, the concepts of improved water and improved sanitation remain controversial. For the purpose of this, and subsequent chapters, the WHO/UNICEF definitions of improved water and improved sanitation are used. The chapter paints a vivid picture of the West and Central Africa region before delving further into the issue of improved water and sanitation.

## The West and Central Africa region

This region extends from the Democratic Republic of Congo in the east/south-east to Mauritania in the west/north-west. It has been described as the world's poorest region (UNICEF, Online). Some 175 million people in this region or half of its entire population lack access to safe drinking water (Ibid). The region can be divided into two sub-regions comprising the mostly Anglophone Western Africa and the almost completely Francophone Central Africa.

*Western Africa*

This sub-region includes sixteen sovereign nations. A majority of these nations were under the colonial tutelage of France. Eight of them, Benin (formerly, Dahomey), Burkina Faso (formerly, Upper Volta), Côte d'Ivoire, Guinea, Mali (formerly, French Sudan), Mauritania, Niger, and Senegal, belonged to a politico-administrative unit, which colonial authorities christened the Federation of French West Africa. This unit was headquartered in the Senegalese capital of Dakar. Togo, an erstwhile colony of Germany, came under French control as a Trust Territory of the League of Nations after World War I. Five of the countries, Ghana, Gambia, Sierra Leone, and Nigeria are former colonies of Britain. Guinea Bissau, and Cape Verde are former colonies of Portugal. Spanish Western Sahara was colonized by Spain. However, Western Sahara has been under the control of Morocco until recently. Liberia is the only country in the region that was never formally colonized. Some knowledge of the colonial background of these countries is crucial for appreciating the nature of their sanitation problematic. This is because their sanitation infrastructure developed around a nucleus developed by colonial powers.

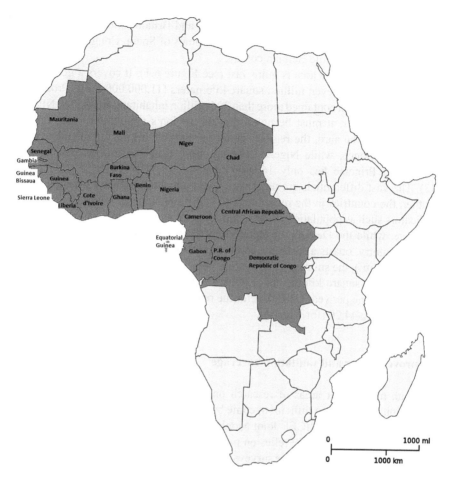

**Figure 6.1 Map of West and Central Africa region**

*Source*: Author's rendition based on blank map from the 'freely-licensed educational media content' world wide website, Wikimedia Commons at http://commons.wikimedia.rg/wiki/category:blank_maps_of_Africa.

*Central Africa*

This sub-region contains eight sovereign countries. Four of these countries, including Chad, Central African Republic (formerly, Ubangi Shari), Gabon and Congo (PRC), are erstwhile French colonies. They constituted the French colonial confederation which went under the name French Equatorial Africa (headquartered in Brazzaville in the People's Republic of Congo). One of the countries, namely Cameroon (formerly, Kamerun) was a German colony. Subsequent to the outcome of World War I, the League of Nations placed Cameroon under the colonial tutelage of France (four-fifths of the territory) and Britain (one-fifth). Equatorial Guinea, and Sao Tome and Principe were colonies of Spain. Congo (Democratic Republic) is an erstwhile Belgian colony.

Taken together, the area is quite vast (see Figure 6.1). It covers a geographic area of more than eleven million square kilometers (11,000,000 km²) (ProInvest, Online). The region contained more than 396 million inhabitants in 2005 (UNICEF, Online). However, it must be noted that the region's population is not evenly distributed. To be sure, the region contains countries that vary tremendously in size. For instance, while Nigeria contains more than 151 million people, Sao Tome and Principe has only 160,000 inhabitants (WHO/UNICEF, 2010: 47-48). The vast differentials are not only associated with the region's demography. Rather, the countries in the region tend to vary tremendously with respect to key indicators such as population density, surface area, and economic endowment. For instance, while the Democratic Republic of Congo, the region's geographically largest country, boasts a surface area of more than two million square kilometers (2,344,900km²), the smallest country, Sao Tome and Principe, has an area of only one thousand square kilometers (1,000km²) (CIA, Online). Similarly, the gross national income per year GNI/Year for the region ranges from 0.10 (for Sao Tome & Principe) to 44.20 (for Nigeria).

## Improved water and sanitation coverage

As with many other areas of research on Africa, accurate and reliable data on sanitation coverage are difficult to come by. The most reliable source of these data to date is the WHO/UNICEF Joint Monitoring Programme (JMP). However, it is important to note that JMP relies on nationally representative household surveys and censuses for its data. These surveys and censuses are conducted under disparate conditions, including varying degrees of geographic accessibility and political constraints. These conditions invariably affect the accuracy and validity of the data. Furthermore, the JMP database includes data from secondary sources such as the International Household Survey Network (IHSN). This renders comparability difficult and sometimes meaningless.

To be sure, the JMP does a fine job to frequently update its data base. While this is commendable, it is sometimes a source of confusion. For instance, the data on sanitation coverage contained in its summary of statistics on "Water, Sanitation and Health (WASH) in West and Central Africa" differ from those appearing in its "Progress on Sanitation and Drinking Water: 2010 Update" (see WHO/UNICEF, 2010; WHO/UNICEF, 2008). The following case in point is illustrative. The sanitation coverage for Central African Republic for 2008 is reported as 31 per cent in the former document (p. 6), and as 34 per cent in the latter (p. 40). Granting, the latter document is presented as an 'update' implying that the data contained therein supersede those appearing in previous publications. However, a researcher without access to the 2010 publication is likely to treat the 2008 version as current and accurate. Nevertheless, it is worth noting that the difference between data in the initial and updated versions is minute. Here, it is important to note that the JMP always issues a cautionary note on all its published data. For instance, in the 2008 document afore-referenced, it cautions that because data are revised for each report, the reports are not comparable (WHO/UNICEF, 2008: 34).

As observed earlier, the West and Central Africa region is comprised of disparate nations that vary in many respects. Paradoxically, this variation is absent when it comes to sanitation coverage. Rather, sanitation conditions throughout the entire region uniformly leave much to be desired. As the United Nations Children's Fund (UNICEF) West and Central Africa Regional Office (WACARO) has noted, the region has the lowest improved sanitation coverage in the world. Only 27 per cent of the region's population has access to improved sanitation facilities (WACARO, Online). This translates to only 105 million people. Therefore, as many as 291 million inhabitants of the region are without access to such facilities. Among the many consequences of this deplorable state of affairs is the fact that, as many as 169 babies of every 1,000 live births die (UNICEF, Online). This is the highest for any major region. A disaggregation of the international statistics on sanitation and related development indicators is very revelatory. For instance, some evidence suggests that poor sanitation conditions in concert with unsafe drinking water are at the root of many preventable deaths resulting from diarrhea, cholera, dysentery, and related ailments in the region (UNICEF, Online). Box 6.1 summarizes sanitation problems and their health consequences for Douala, Cameroon's premier commercial city, and one of the largest cities in the region.

**Box 6.1 Sanitation conditions in Douala, Cameroon**

Douala is Cameroon's premier commercial city. It has a population of almost 2.5 million. Sanitation conditions are generally poor in most parts of the city, especially the densely populated low-income neighbourhoods of New Bell, Bepanda, Brazzaville, Madagascar and Quartier Nylon.

The city has no central sewerage system. Thus, the few households that can afford it have private septic tanks. The impoverished majority use pit latrines or defecate in the open. The high density and congested nature of residential areas in especially the ultra-low-income areas means that latrines and areas of open defecation are typically close to water wells. In fact, the poor management of human and domestic waste is commonplace in especially the slum districts of the city. Here domestic wastewater is evacuated indiscriminately. This ends up creating standing pools of filthy water that discharge pungent odours into the air. The situation is aggravated by natural environmental factors. Prominent among these factors are: sandy soil, vast expanses of swamps, high water table, algae-infested ditches and rivers, and frequent flooding. These factors facilitate transmission of raw sewage and untreated domestic wastes. In addition, wastewater from industries, hospitals and other facilities is discharged directly into the environment. Some recent studies of sanitation in the city have uncovered evidence attesting to the presence of effluents rich in coliforms, faecal matter, helminthes, viruses, protozoa and various chemical and physical pollutants (Ndjama et al., 2008). Man-made problems such as overcrowding and uncontrolled urbanization are also high on the list of factors contributing to the health and sanitation quandary of Douala.

*Source*: Author's field research notes.

The sanitation coverage for the region differs markedly between urban and rural areas. While 34 per cent of the population in urban areas has access to improved sanitation facilities, only 17 per cent of those living in rural areas are served by similar facilities (WHO/UNICEF, 2008: 7). The pronounced urban-rural disparity in sanitation coverage noted for the West and Central Africa region is not unique. Rather, it is a worldwide phenomenon. In fact, seven out of every 10 people without access to improved sanitation in the world live in a rural area (WHO/UNICEF, 2008: 16). This disparity is even more dramatic when one considers the progress in access to improved sanitation that has been made since the 1990s. In this regard, 64 per cent of the 1.3 billion people who gained access to improved sanitation worldwide between 1990 and 2008 live in urban areas (Ibid: 17).

In the West and Central Africa region, only one country, namely Gambia, boasts improved sanitation coverage of more than 50 per cent for rural areas (see Table 6.1). In fact, the Gambian case, with 65 per cent sanitation coverage for rural areas, is an anomaly. It is arguably a function of the country's colonial legacy. The resident European population in Gambia during the colonial era was relatively small. In contrast to what obtained elsewhere in colonial West and Central Africa, Europeans were not concentrated in one area of the colonial capital. In addition, members of the indigenous population had vehemently and successfully fought to prevent racial residential segregation throughout Gambia. This, among other things, meant that colonial authorities could not concentrate sanitation infrastructure development efforts in one specific area. Rather, it was necessary to provide some level of improved sanitation throughout the Gambian territory in order to serve members of the dispersed European population.

Other countries in the region had a completely different colonial experience. Racial residential segregation was the norm, and improved sanitation and other public services were provided exclusively in European enclaves of colonial towns. Most of the cities with populations of one million or more in the region originated as colonial cities. These cities have experienced rapid rates of population growth during the last two decades. At the same time the rural populations have been shrinking. Yet, throughout the region, according to published data, improvements in sanitation conditions have progressed faster in urban, than in rural, areas. In 2006, it was reported that only one country, Gambia, in the West Africa sub-region had urban sanitation coverage greater than 50 per cent (Awuah, 2009: 5). However, as Table 6.1 shows, the situation has improved markedly over the course of just two years. The most recent data from JMP indicate that urban coverage in four countries in the West Africa sub-region, including Senegal (69%), Gambia (68%), and Cape Verde (65%), have now reached or exceeded 50 per cent. However, only one country, Cameroon (56%) in the central Africa sub-region has attained or exceeded the 50 per cent mark for improved sanitation coverage in urban areas. In contrast, progress in access to improved sanitation in rural areas has been very slow. As noted earlier, with the exception of Gambia, no country in the region has a coverage level for improved sanitation in excess of 50 per cent in rural areas. Many countries, Burkina Faso, Chad, Ghana, Liberia, Niger, and Sierra Leone, in the region have coverage levels for sanitation in rural areas of less than 10 per cent.

On the whole, water and sanitation conditions tend to be better in erstwhile colonial cities than elsewhere in the region. The reason for this is simple. Colonial authorities did everything in their power to ensure that Europeans in Africa enjoyed sanitation and other conditions comparable to what obtained in European towns at the time. When the colonial era ended, the former exclusively European enclaves along with the sanitation and concomitant infrastructure were inherited by indigenous elites. This provides at least partial explanation for the fact that sanitation conditions are better in urban areas than their rural counterparts.

Another question worth addressing has to do with the fact that sanitation conditions are better in some cities in the region than in others. Even more puzzling is the fact that marked differences in water and sanitation conditions exist among towns with identical backgrounds within the same country. Two opposite cases in point are worth noting.

Table 6.1 Water and sanitation coverage for West and Central Africa, 2008

| Country | Total Population (1000s) | Surface area (km²) | Percent urban population | Improved sanitation coverage (%) | | Improved water coverage (%) | |
|---|---|---|---|---|---|---|---|
| | | | | Urban | Rural | Urban | Rural |
| Benin | 8662 | 112,622 | 41 | 24 | 4 | 84 | 69 |
| Burkina Faso | 15234 | 274,200 | 20 | 33 | 6 | 95 | 72 |
| Cameroon | 19088 | 475,440 | 57 | 56 | 35 | 92 | 51 |
| Cape Verde | 499 | 4,033 | 60 | 65 | 38 | 85 | 82 |
| C. African Rep. | 4339 | 622,984 | 39 | 43 | 28 | 92 | 51 |
| Chad | 10914 | 1,284,000 | 27 | 23 | 4 | 67 | 44 |
| Congo (DR) | 64257 | 2,344,858 | 34 | 23 | 23 | 80 | 28 |
| Congo (PR) | 3615 | 342,000 | 61 | 31 | 29 | 95 | 34 |
| Cote d'Ivoire | 20591 | 322,462 | 49 | 36 | 11 | 93 | 68 |
| Equatorial Guinea | 659 | 28,051 | 39 | – | – | – | – |
| Gabon | 1448 | 267,667 | 85 | 33 | 30 | 95 | 41 |
| Gambia | 1660 | 11,295 | 57 | 68 | 65 | 96 | 86 |
| Ghana | 23351 | 238,500 | 50 | 18 | 7 | 90 | 74 |
| Guinea | 9833 | 255,857 | 34 | 34 | 11 | 89 | 61 |
| Guinea Bissau | 1575 | 36,125 | 30 | 49 | 9 | 83 | 51 |
| Liberia | 3793 | 99,067 | 60 | 25 | 4 | 79 | 51 |
| Mali | 12706 | 1,240,192 | 32 | 45 | 32 | 81 | 44 |
| Mauritania | 3215 | 1,031,00 | 41 | 50 | 9 | 52 | 47 |
| Niger | 14704 | 1,267,000 | 16 | 34 | 4 | 96 | 39 |
| Nigeria | 151212 | 923,768 | 48 | 36 | 28 | 75 | 42 |
| S.Tome/Principe | 160 | 964 | 61 | 30 | 19 | 89 | 88 |
| Senegal | 12211 | 196,722 | 42 | 69 | 38 | 92 | 52 |
| Sierra Leone | 5560 | 72,740 | 38 | 24 | 6 | 86 | 26 |
| Togo | 6459 | 56,785 | 42 | 24 | 3 | 87 | 41 |

*Source*: WHO/UNICEF (2010) available online at: http://www.who.int/water_sanitation_health/monitoring/fast_facts/en/index.html. Figures on surface area are from the US CIA Factbook: https://www.cia.gov/library/publications/the-world-factbook/wfExt/region_afr.html.

On the one hand there is Accra, Ghana. Accra with a population of almost two million (1,963,264), is Ghana's capital city (Boardi, 2004). Water and sanitation conditions in the city are generally better than what obtains in many capital cities throughout West Africa. Water scarcity is hardly an issue in this city. In fact, three major sources of water, including the Kpong system on the Volta River, the Weija system on the Densu River and the Boso system, are available to the city. Most of the city's residents use water from formal water supply systems, including pipe borne and vendours. About 49 per cent of the population has water on-site, that is, within their plot of land. Ten per cent boasts indoor plumbing, 39 per cent has yard connection, 22 per cent depends on water from neighbours, while 16 per cent depend on vendours to meet their water needs. A substantial portion of the city's population fetches water from public standpipes.

Sanitation conditions in Accra also tend to be systematically better than one is likely to find in other African cities. For instance, public toilets, which are scarce to non-existent in other African cities, are readily available in Accra. This notwithstanding, it is important to note that the distribution of sanitation is very uneven, and skewed in favour of middle- and upper-income districts throughout the city. Consequently, the low income residential areas tend to be terribly underserved. As much as 37 per cent of the urban population in Ghana has no indoor toilet facilities. Of these, 35 per cent rely on public toilets and about three per cent (2.5%) defecate in the open (Boadi, 2004).

On the other hand, there is Bamako, the capital city of Mali (Brinkhoff, 2010; WSUP, 2009). In contrast to Accra, Bamako suffers from a shortage of water. The city is largely flat and arid. Thus, water supply is highly limited in this city. The city depends on one source, the Niger River, to meet its water needs. According to the United Nations Environment Programme (UNEP), this means extra expenditures for the municipal authorities as they must see into it that the water is treated and ready for consumption. Although the river typically runs very shallow most of the year, during periods of intensive rainfall, it tends to overflow its banks. Resulting from this have often been floods with significant health consequences. There have been aggressive efforts in recent times to drain this flat inland city with the installation of improved storm water drainage systems and solid waste management programmes (Brinkhoff, 2010).

On the whole, Bamako has a safe sanitation coverage level of about 28 per cent (WSUP, 2009). Like most cities in the West and Central Africa region, the city has no central sewerage system. The United Nations Centre for Human Settlements (UN-Habitat) (2006) noted that the city has three networks of mini-sewers of 38.5 km and nine small hidden sanitation canals of about 27 km. This limited sanitation infrastructure serves only one to two per cent of the city's population. The mini-sewers are designed to handle grey water as opposed to human wastes. Sanitation at the household level typically involves the use of latrines. Latrines are anything but uniform. Rather, they come in different varieties. About 15 per cent of households in low-income districts use latrines with wood slabs, while the majority (85%) uses simple latrines with concrete slabs. Only a very small minority uses flush toilets that discharge into individual household septic tanks (Debomey, 2003).

## Institutional frameworks

Institutional frameworks are of centrality in the discourse on water and sanitation. An understanding of these frameworks can enhance our knowledge of barriers and opportunities in the water and sanitation sector. The frameworks constitute the formal laws, regulations and procedures that govern the operations of agencies responsible for delivering water, sanitation and related services. Their importance is heightened in the West and Central Africa region because of their unique history and the evolutionary process they have undergone. Water, hygiene and sanitation were not recognized as inextricably intertwined services until several decades subsequent to the official onset of the colonial era in the region. Prior to that, the production, storage and delivery of water were undertaken on a small scale. Services were limited exclusively to European enclaves. As for hygiene and sanitation, these were regarded as matters that could be handled at the household level.

Developments in Europe, particularly advancements in knowledge of contagious diseases contributed to changing this line of thinking. This led to colonial governments assuming responsibility for the promotion and protection of public health. Accordingly, units of government were created throughout most of the colonies and placed in charge of water supply. Hygiene and sanitation, by default, fell under the auspices of public health departments. This is because no specific unit of government was established to directly take care of sanitation and hygiene matters. If water had risen to the top of the agenda of colonial governments it is because of its paramount role in facilitating other aspects of sanitation. Water is necessary for cleaning and operating modern sanitation facilities. In the British colonies of the region it was common to place the responsibility for water supply under the Public Works Department (PWD). This was the case in British Southern Cameroons (now, the Anglophone area of Cameroon), Nigeria, and Ghana. The Ghanaian case, summarized in Box 6.2, epitomizes the evolution of thinking on water and sanitation as basic services in the region.

One noteworthy piece of information that can be gleaned from the box is the extent to which the institutional arrangement for water and sanitation has changed over time in Ghana. Also worth noting is the fact that responsibility for water and sanitation has always been fragmented. To be sure, the Ghanaian case is not unique in both regards. In fact, the region's Francophone countries appear to have experienced more changes in the sanitation and water sector than their Anglophone counterparts. Consider the case of Cameroon whose administrative structure has been wholly influenced by French politico-administrative philosophy despite the fact that it is one-fifth Anglophone. Here, as Box 6.3 shows, the first formal government entity in charge of water was created in 1952. This entity, the

Agricultural Engineering Department *(Service du Génie Rural)* of the Ministry of Agriculture was responsible for supplying water to rural areas in the northern part of the country.

## Box 6.2 Evolution of water and sanitation sector in Ghana

In Ghana, a formal government entity in charge of water supply was created as far back as 1928. This entity, the Hydraulics Unit of the Public Works Department (PWD), was responsible for water supply. However, its services were limited to urban areas. Twenty years later in 1948, another unit, the Rural Water Department was created within PWD and charged with the responsibility of rural water supply. In 1958, the urban and rural water supply units of PWD merged to become the Water Supply Division of PWD. All this while, the responsibility for sanitation was under the jurisdiction of a separate government unit. It was not until 1965 that water and at least one aspect of sanitation, namely sewerage, came under the same institutional umbrella, the Ghana Water and Sewerage Corporation (GWSC). In 1994 urban and rural water supply services were once more separated with the creation of the Community Water and Sanitation Department of GWSC. Since then, the water and sanitation sector in Ghana has witnessed several institutional reform actions. Presently, the sector includes government entities, national and international non-governmental organizations (NGOs), and private corporations, such as Acqua Vitens Rand.

*Source*: Adapted from UNICEF (Online).

The northern region of Cameroon has scarcely any rivers and is characterized by rugged terrain and extremely dry soil. This partially explains its selection as the focus of early colonial government water supply initiatives. A decade later, and one year after independence, an administrative reform action in Cameroon resulted in the creation of the Office of Water within the Ministry of Transport, Mines and Telecommunications (*Ministère des Transports, des Mines et des Télécommunications*). This entity was given the specific charge of exploring ground water as well as conducting inventories of water points. This has since been followed by a series of further reform initiatives that have culminated in at least fifteen major changes in the water and sanitation sector. The most recent of these changes took place under Decree No. 2010/0239/PM in 2010. It entailed transferring the management of wells and boreholes to local communes while placing the responsibility for potable water networks under the state. Five years earlier, in 2005, Decree No. 2005/494 had created the Cameroon Water Utilities Corporation (CAMWATER). This was part of initiatives designed to privatize the water and sanitation sector. These initiatives resulted in the privatization of the Cameroon Water Corporation (*Société Nationale d'Eaux du Cameroun*) in 2008.

## Box 6.3 Major institutional reforms in the water and sanitation sector in Cameroon

1952: First government unit in charge of water is created. The unit, the Agricultural Engineering Department *(Service du Génie Rural)* was established as part of the Ministry of Agriculture and placed in charge of rural water supply in the northern part of the country.

1962: The Office of Water is created within the Ministry of Transport, Mines and Telecommunications *(Ministère des Transports, des Mines et des Télécommunications)*. It was placed in charge of exploring ground water and inventorying water points.

1968: The National Water Supply Company of Cameroon *(SNEC: Société Nationale des Eaux du Cameroun)* is created. It was given the charge of operating urban water supply networks in the country for 40 years.

1977: The Ministry of Mines and Energy *(Ministère des Mines et de l'Énergie)*, is placed in charge of urban water and sanitation services while the responsibility for rural water supply was retained under the Ministry of Agriculture.

1984: Law No. 084/013, stipulating water regulations, is enacted.

1988: The Ministry of Mines and Energy is re-organized and re-named, the Ministry of Mines, Energy and Water *(Ministère des Mines, de l'Énergie et de l'Eau)*. It becomes the ministerial body in charge of water and sanitation services throughout the entire country. The Directorate of Rural Water Supply *(DHR: Direction de l'Hydraulique Rurale)* is placed in charge of rural water supply while the Directorate of Urban Water and Sanitation *(DEAU: Direction de l'Eau et de l'Assainissement Urbain)* is placed in charge of urban water supply and sanitation.

1992: Law No. 92-002 pertaining to the creation of communes (local authorities) is enacted.

1996: DHR and DEAU are merged to form the Directorate of Water *(DE: Direction de l'Eau)* in charge of water and sanitation services in rural and urban towns.

1998: A new law (No. 98/005) pertaining to water regulations is supplemented by implementing provisions, as of 2001, that also pertain to the management of the service.

1999: Start of the SNEC privatization process (limited Invitation to Tender for 51 per cent of shares).

2000: Provisional acquisition of SNEC by the French utility company, 'Suez Lyonnaise des Eaux' (ONDEO Services).

2002: Nomination of a temporary administrator to oversee the privatization process and ensure continuity of the public water service.

2003: Admission that acquisition of SNEC by ONDEO Services has failed, announcement of a new means of privatization that is still being defined.

2004: Law No. 2004/18 setting out the rules applicable to communes.

2005: Decree No. 2005/493 setting out the means of delegation of WSS public services in urban and peri-urban areas. Decree No. 2005/494 pertaining to the creation of the Cameroon Water Utilities Corporation (CAMWATER).

2008: Conclusion of the SNEC privatization process with the establishment of a leasing contract for the management and operation of urban facilities between the state, Camwater, and Camerounaise des Eaux (subsidiary of ONEP, national water supply company of Morocco).

2010: Decree No. 2010/0239/PM transferring the construction and management of wells and boreholes to communes (the drinking water networks remain with the state).

*Source*: UNICEF (Online).

A perusal of the institutional frameworks for water and sanitation policy administration in West and Central Africa reveals a number of factors that are capable of stifling their functioning. One of these factors, which is discernible from the example of Ghana (Box 6.2) and that of Cameroon (Box 6.3), has to do with the frequency of institutional re-organization. One can appreciate the need for reforms necessary to keep abreast with changing times. However, when reforms are initiated with the frequency noted here, their benefits are often dwarfed by their demerits. The demerits are easy to understand. Institutional reforms entail the commitment of precious time to logistical matters, re-organizing office space and developing new working relationships, among other things. This is time that would have otherwise gone towards actually crafting and/or implementing water and sanitation policies.

Another attribute of the institutional frameworks for water and sanitation in the region is their proclivity for fragmentation. In this regard, responsibility for water, hygiene and sanitation is often distributed among several, sometimes disparate, entities. For instance, Burkina Faso's 2008 public institutional reform initiative culminated in among other things, the separation of water and sanitation management. In the rural areas, this separation was effectively accomplished with the establishment of the General Directorate of Wastewater, Sanitation and Human Excreta (*DGAEUE: Direction Générale de l'Assainissement des Eaux Usées et Excrétas*). The equivalence of this in the urban areas was the creation of the General Directorate of Water Resources (*DGRE: Direction Générale des Ressources en Eau*). The problem is rendered more difficult by the increasing wave of privatization initiatives that have occurred or are ongoing throughout Africa as a whole. As Box 6.3 shows, Cameroon's water privatization efforts were concluded in 2008. This is when the country's national water corporation moved from the public to the private sphere.

Actors in the water and sanitation policy field in countries in the region now include entities from all sectors. In this case, the national actors include, the main government ministerial bodies involved in the water and sanitation sector either as direct suppliers or overseers (see Table 6.2). Sub-national entities include the regional units of ministerial bodies and municipal governments. In addition, there are international and local non-governmental organizations (NGOs), which are also active in the field. The international NGOs are involved mainly in technical advisory capacities or funding sources. In addition, there are community organizations that bring together citizens to complete local water and sanitation projects as self-help initiatives. With this multitude of entities, coordination invariably ranks high among the challenges confronting water and sanitation authorities in the region.

**Table 6.2 Government ministries in charge of water and sanitation in Africa**

| Country | Government Ministeries in Charge of Water and Sanitation |
|---|---|
| Benin | 1) Ministry of Energy, Water & Mines; 2) Ministry of Environment, Housing & Urban Development; 3) Ministry of Health. |
| Burkina Faso | 1) Ministry of Agriculture, Water & Fisheries; 2) Ministry of Housing & Urbanization; 3) Ministry of Health. |
| Cameroon | 1) Ministry of Energy & Water Resources; 2) Ministry of Urban Development & Housing; 3) Ministry of Public Health. |
| Cape Verde | 1) Ministry of Environment, Housing & Territorial Administration; 2) Ministry of Health. |
| C. African Rep. | 1) Ministry of Public Health; 2) Ministry of Transport & Equipment. |
| Chad | 1) Ministry of Urban Planning & Housing; 2) Ministry of Water; 3) Ministry of Public Health. |
| Congo (DR) | 1) Ministry of Infrastructure, Public Works & Reconstruction; 2) Ministry of Urban Planning & Housing; 3) Ministry of Health. |
| Congo (PR) | 1) Ministry of Construction, Town Planning & Housing; 2) Ministry of Energy & Water; 3) Ministry of Health. |
| Cote d'Ivoire | 1) Ministry of Livestock, Water Resources & Fisheries; 2) Ministry of Planning & Development. |
| Equatorial Guinea | 1) Ministry of Health & Social Welfare; 2) Ministry of Public Works & Infrastructure. |
| Gabon | 1) Ministry of State for Housing & Town Planning; 2) Ministry of Forests, Water & Fishing Economy; 2) Ministry of Public Health & Sanitation in charge of Family & Promotion of Women. |
| Gambia | 1) Ministry of Fisheries, Water Resources and National Assembly; 2) Ministry of Health & Social Welfare; 3) Ministry of Works, Construction & Infrastructure. |
| Ghana | 1) Ministry of Health; Ministry of Water Resources, Works & Housing. |
| Guinea | 1) Ministry of Urbanism, Habitat & Construction; 2) Ministry of Public Works; 3) Ministry of Health & Public Hygiene. |
| Guinea Bissau | 1) Ministry of Health; 2) Ministry of Infrastructure, Transport & Communication. |
| Liberia | 1) Ministry of Health & Social Welfare; 2) Ministry of Public Works. |

| Mali | 1) Ministry of Environment & Sanitation; 2) Ministry of Energy & Water Resources; 3) Ministry of Housing, Land Affairs & Town Development. |
|---|---|
| Mauritania | 1) Ministry of Habitat, Urban Affairs, & Territorial Administration; 2) Ministry of Health; 3) Ministry of Hydrology & Sanitation. |
| Niger | 1) Ministry of Health; 2) Ministry of Urban Development, Housing & Sanitation; 3) Ministry of Water Resources. |
| Nigeria | 1) Federal Ministry of Health; 2) Federal Ministry of Agriculture & Water Resources. |
| Sao Tome & Principe | 1) Ministry of Health; 2) Ministry of Public Works & Infrastructure, Urban Development, Transportation & Communications. |
| Senegal | 1) Ministry of Urbanism, Sanitation, Public Hygiene & Quality of Life; 2) Ministry of Health & Prevention; 3) Ministry of State for Urban Development, Housing, Hydraulics & Sanitation. |
| Siera Leone | 1) Ministry of Health & Sanitation; 2) Ministry of Lands, Country Planning & Environment; 2) Ministry of Works, Housing & Infrastructural Development. |
| Togo | 1) Ministry of Health; 2) Ministry of Planning & Housing. |

*Source*:   https://www.cia.gov/library/publications/world-leaders-1/   and   http://www.commonwealth-of-nations.org.

## Constraints to improving hygiene and sanitation conditions

The West and Central Africa region is saddled with so many problems that make improving its hygiene and sanitation conditions an uphill battle. Prominent in this regard is the problem of poverty, which is a defining characteristic of the region. The region is home to some of the poorest countries, including Liberia, Niger, Sierra Leone, and Togo, which had an estimated GDP per capita of less than $1,000 in 2010 (CIA, Online). More than half of the population of almost all countries in the region lives on less than one US dollar a day. By established UN standards, this means that more than half of the region's population is extremely poor. Poverty and poor hygiene and sanitation conditions are reciprocally related. Without financial resources, households cannot afford the materials and skilled labour necessary to improve their hygiene and sanitation conditions. The lack of improved hygiene conditions causes diseases that often weaken the economic productive capacity of people, thereby rendering them poor. Yet, the importance of sanitation is not limited to its indisputable contribution to economic productivity. In fact, sanitation constitutes a critical element in efforts to attain the millennium development goals (MDGs). Sanitation possesses the potential to contribute significantly to efforts to promote gender equity. The UNICEF/WHO Joint Monitoring Programme (JMP) summarizes the importance of sanitation to development in general more succinctly in the following terms. Sanitation: "is vital for human health; generates economic benefits; contributes to dignity and social development; and helps the environment" (Awuah, 2009: 4).

Another critical factor that cannot be ignored in discussions of constraints to efforts to improve hygiene and sanitation conditions in the region is nature. The contributions to poverty or wealth of natural factors, such as the availability or lack of natural resources constitute the subject of many socio-political and economic discussions. Less frequently discussed, however, is the impact of these factors on hygiene and sanitation. Yet, natural conditions have been known to stifle efforts to improve hygiene and sanitation conditions in the West and Central African region. Consider the case of Cameroon, a country that has enjoyed political stability since independence. Here, initiatives to provide potable water to residents of the country's northern region have been derailed by difficult weather and geological conditions. The region is characterized by extended dry seasons, rugged terrain and very hard soil. Typically, people, animals and birds must use the few available watering holes. Schools in the region often go without water points or latrines. According to UNICEF (2005), these conditions have often been at the root of epidemics of cholera and meningitis in the region. This phenomenon is commonplace throughout the Sahel zone, which circumscribes countries such as Chad, Niger, Burkina Faso, and Mali. In some of these countries, the problem is not one of complete wetness or dryness. Rather, it is typically an extreme case of one or the other. For example, in Chad, during some parts of the year, the south experiences high torrential rainfall. This often causes a rise in water tables and unbearable floods. The eastern part of the same country is extremely rocky and dry, thereby making it difficult to dig water wells. The central and northern part of the country is sandy. Ordinarily, this will imply less difficulty in digging water wells. However, the water table in this region is extremely deep.

Efforts to improve hygiene and sanitation conditions in the West and Central Africa region have also been significantly constrained by man-made catastrophes, especially war. Five countries in the region, including Chad, Côte d'Ivoire, Liberia, Sierra Leone and the Democratic Republic of Congo, have witnessed their scant inventory of water and sanitation infrastructure devastated by civil war. Basic services, including electricity, water and sanitation constitute a casualty of armed conflicts in these countries. Even where such conflicts have ended, reinstating these services has proven to be an insurmountable task to the resource-strapped post-war governments. Chad has had a series of prolonged civil wars for more than four decades (1965 to 2010). Apart from rendering any government effort to develop new water and sanitation facilities, the war destroyed most of the infrastructure that had been developed by colonial authorities. To compound the problem, the country's meager sanitation infrastructure has been overtaxed in the recent past by refugees escaping violent conflicts in neighboring Darfur.

Côte d'Ivoire's civil war that began in 2002 had far-reaching implications for public health throughout the country. According to UNICEF (Online), more than 85 per cent of the medical personnel in opposition-held zones abandoned their posts during the conflict. To worsen matters, no less than 70 per cent of the country's medical facilities were closed due to the civil war. Although calm has recently returned to the country, the reverberating effects of the war remain very visible in its water and sanitation infrastructure and health statistics. In this latter regard, there has been a significant increase in vulnerability to epidemics, preventable diseases and malnutrition (UNICEF, Online). In addition, a number of the health facilities that were shut down by the war have not been re-opened. Furthermore, many of the water and sanitation systems that were destroyed by the war are yet to, or may never, be repaired.

In Liberia, fourteen years of civil war (1989–2003) resulted in the destruction of a significant segment of the country's water and sanitation infrastructure. In addition, the war displaced at least 500,000 people (UNICEF, Online). Most of the internally displaced persons continue to live in camps, with very little in the way of hygiene and sanitation facilities. A good many have since made permanent homes in slum settlements, which are equally devoid of such facilities. Neighbouring Sierra Leone suffered an eleven-year bloody civil war (1991–2002) which wreaked havoc on the country's human settlements. The inattention to water and sanitation infrastructure during the war resulted in permanent damage to the system. Although the war ended almost a decade ago, things are yet to return to normalcy. The re-established civil administration is strapped for cash, and has very limited avenues for income generation. This has rendered difficult any efforts to build new infrastructure and facilities or repair existing ones.

The devastating effects of civil war on hygiene and sanitation can also be seen in Kivu in eastern Congo (DR). Here, civil war displaced almost a million people in the region. In addition, it resulted in the destruction of sanitation and water services in major towns such as Lubero in North Kivu. Oxfam and other international NGOs have since been working to prevent the loss of lives in the region. In particular, Oxfam and her partners have been responsible for trucking 200,000 litres of potable water every day to people in the affected towns (Oxfam, Online). The devastation of the war is more pronounced once one appreciates the fact that the Democratic Republic of Congo is one of the nations most endowed with water on earth. The world renowned River Congo and a lot of smaller rivers crisscross the Congolese countryside. On their own, these rivers constitute great sources of natural water. However, more than a decade of war has displaced people, rendered once safe and lush country sides too dangerous for everyone, including the native inhabitants. The only safe havens in the country are the major cities and temporary camps operated by international NGOs. These camps are breeding grounds for lethal but preventable diseases, including but not limited to diarrhea, dysentery, cholera, and pneumonia.

The sanitation picture of the West and Central Africa region can be better appreciated by closely examining some of the region's largest cities. Accordingly, we now turn our focus to three of the most populous cities in region, namely Abidjan, Kinshasa and Lagos.

### Sanitation issues in Abidjan, Côte d'Ivoire

With a population of 3.8 million (UN-Habitat, 2009), Abidjan qualifies as the sub-region's second largest city. It was the colonial government capital of Côte d'Ivoire from 1931 until the country gained political independence from France in 1960. It served as that country's administrative capital until 1983 when it ceded its place as the administrative capital to Yamoussoukro. With a population of 3.8 million (UNdata, Online), Abidjan remains Côte d'Ivoire's largest and most commercially active city. It is the second largest city in West Africa after Lagos, Nigeria, and the fourth largest French-speaking city in the world after Paris, France; Montreal, Canada, and Kinshasa, Congo (DR).

Abidjan is a coastal city situated on a lagoon, the Ebrié Lagoon, which sits on several converging peninsulas and islands that are linked by bridges. As a low-lying locale, the city is prone to flooding. The most affected districts in this connection are Yopougon and Abobo. The city is amongst the most industrialized and densely populated in West Africa. This means, among other things, that it wrestles with some of the most intense environmental problems in the region. Wastes from industrial activities such as petroleum, chemical, textile, wood and food processing are typically discharged directly into the ocean or open fields (Huton et al., 2007). This indiscriminate disposal of industrial waste has severe consequences for the health of the city's residents.

Yet, available evidence suggests that Abidjan is considerably well-served by sanitation facilities in comparison to other cities in the West African region. However, it bears noting that only 10 to 35 per cent of the city's population, most of them based in the wealthy and middle-income districts, is connected to standard sanitation facilities (Collignon et al., 2000). The majority of the population depends on low-quality sanitation facilities, including bucket latrines, improved pit latrines, and toilets that empty into onsite septic tanks (Ibid). Nationally, according to some estimates, 20 to 30 per cent of the urban population in Côte d'Ivoire has access to improved sanitation facilities (UNICEF and WCARO, 2008). By other estimates, as much as 61 per cent of the urban population and 23 per cent of those in rural areas have access to improved sanitation services and facilities (UNICEF, Online). The remainder of the population resorts to using rudimentary sanitation facilities, while a significant proportion practices open defecation.

With respect to sewerage, Abidjan ranks higher than most cities in the West Africa sub-region. In this regard, the city boasts an extensive drainage and sewerage system that was developed in the 1970s and 1980s. Developed with the financial support of the World Bank, this system comprises a main collector of 23 kilometers, a network of 640 kilometers, and as many as 45 installations (Collignon et al., 2000). The installations include pumping and pretreatment stations. This extensive network covers many areas within the city, including Koumassi, Marcory, Vridi, Treichville, Abobo and Yopougon.

According to the IMF Poverty Reduction Strategy Paper on Côte d'Ivoire, the country has a long way to go to attain adequate sanitation coverage for its population. A logical starting point for success in this regard is to craft sanitation master plans or establish some bench marks to guide sanitation improvement and related initiatives. However, very few municipalities in Côte d'Ivoire have developed such plans or benchmarks. In fact, only seven of the country's major cities have a sanitation master plan. The municipalities include, Abidjan, Bouake, Yamoussoukro, Daoukro, Daloa, Gagnoa, and San-Pedro. Particularly noteworthy here is the fact that the country's premier city, Abidjan tends to be the main, and in some cases, the exclusive focus of sanitation initiatives in the country. For this reason, the city alone is the beneficiary of as much as 2,000 kilometers of piped sewerage network (IMF, 2009: 67). Yet, despite the sanitation infrastructure investment bias in favour of Abidjan, the city's sanitation network suffers from serious neglect and disrepair. As the IMF Poverty Reduction Strategy Paper for the country noted, since 1996 the network, comprising 2,000 km of pipelines and 51 sewage backflow and lift stations, has never benefited from any major maintenance initiative.

Abidjan's annual industrial and household effluents amount to 4.4 million cubic meters. These effluents empty into the Ebrié Lagoon, and tend to contribute significantly to flooding problems in areas around the lagoon. Two communities, Yopougon and Abobo frequently bear the brunt of the flooding. On the whole, most Ivoirians, as the IMF report concludes, do not enjoy environmental hygiene (IMF, 2009: 67). The situation is similar in the sub-region's largest city, Lagos, which is the focus of the next segment.

## The sanitation situation in Lagos, Nigeria

Lagos was the administrative and commercial capital of Nigeria during the colonial era. It maintained this status until 12 December 1991 when the seat of the Nigerian Federal Government was relocated to Abuja. The population of this megacity is estimated to be about 11 million (UN, 2009). This makes Lagos the most populous city in the West Africa sub-region in particular and sub-Saharan Africa in general. With a growth rate of 5 to 10 per cent per annum, Lagos ranks among the fastest growing cities in the world.

Lagos was, and continues to be, the economic nerve center of West Africa. During the colonial era, it boasted water and sanitation facilities that would earn the praises of even the most stoic critic. The facilities ranged from functional street lights to well-manicured public parks and golf courses. The city was the beneficiary of segregationist medical and sanitary measures, which colonial authorities directed exclusively at European districts. With the demise of colonialism, indigenous elites inherited what used to be exclusive European enclaves. Thus, for a few years subsequent to the demise of colonialism, sanitation conditions in Lagos were good. However, with the passage of time, the formerly 'native districts' grew, proliferated and encroached upon the previously exclusively European enclaves. These areas, it must be recalled, were denied access to all sanitation facilities.

Not long after independence, the municipal government witnessed its revenue generating ability wane. At the same time sanitation conditions in the rapidly expanding erstwhile 'native' districts grew worse, while the sanitation facilities in the elite enclaves were growing increasingly in need of maintenance and repairs. Before long, a substantial portion of the facilities had ceased functioning. This was the case especially during the 1970s. In the 1980s, negative trends in the global economy spelt doom for Nigeria. Consequently, municipal governments, including the government of Lagos State all but stopped maintaining existing, let alone supply additional, water and sanitation infrastructure. This, in a nutshell, is how Lagos found itself where it is today with respect to its sanitation infrastructure and condition.

Paradoxically, despite its history as one of the oldest modern cities on the West coast of Africa, Lagos remains without a central wastewater collection system. A number of other relevant statistics paint a grim picture of the water and sanitation situation of this megacity. For purposes of illustration, consider the following (Moe and Rheingans, 2006):

- public water covers only 35 per cent of the metro-population.
- more than 60 per cent of the water is lost due to leakages;
- 65 per cent of the population relies on private water wells;
- 30 per cent of the households use pit latrines;
- 53 per cent of the households use flush or pour-flush toilets;
- less than 12 per cent have access to a working water-borne sanitation systems.

The sanitation problems of Lagos are magnified several folds when juxtaposed with those of other cities in Africa. Some of the problems are of the natural variant while others are man-made. In the former regard, it is worth noting that most of Lagos is comprised of lagoon. Wetlands cover as much as 42 per cent of the area, which is subject to flooding. Most of the land is low-lying, and only 15 meters above sea level on the average. Victoria Island, Lagos/Ikoyi Islands, and Apapa are flat. These natural features render the city highly vulnerable to floods. Also problematic in real and potential terms is the fact that the water table in most of the city is high. Thus, in some areas one needs to dig just three meters into the ground to find water. This would bode well for efforts to meet the city's water needs but for the fact that the water is not drinkable. Additionally, it should be noted that the porosity content of soil in Lagos is very high. This invariably increases the chance of sewage and other wastewater infiltrating and polluting ground water and well water—the source of water in most of the city. When it floods, as it is commonplace in Lagos, sewage and other wastes are carried into water wells.

Some analysts have been rather blunt in characterizing Lagos as the filthiest of all megacities in the world (Adedibu and Okekunle, 1989). Access to improved sanitation facilities is restricted to the upper and middle-income districts of the city. In the poor districts, people must resort to improvising their own means of dealing with domestic and human wastes. Defecating in plastic bags and indiscriminately disposing of same has become popular as an improvised method of human waste collection and disposal. Apart from the scarcity of public toilets, the city lacks a functional waste disposal system. Consequently, large amounts of domestic, industrial and human wastes are left untreated and discharged into the environment (Huton et al., 2007). This has far-reaching implications for environmental pollution and the concomitant spread of infectious diseases.

Over the years, Lagos has significantly grown in demographic and spatial terms. Spatially, the city has grown to encompass areas beyond the lagoon and circumscribing as many as 200 different slums in the vicinity (Gandy, 2006). The slums range in size from clusters of shacks located underneath street and highway bridges, to entire districts such as Ajegunle and Mushin. Concomitant with this growth has been a marked deterioration in sanitation conditions and quality of life. The following specific examples serve to drive this point home (Gandy, 2006):

- Lack of, or malfunctioning, street lights in many parts of the city;
- Rapidly deteriorating and congested streets;
- Lack of, or irregular, refuse collection;
- Rise in violent crime rates;
- Lack of sewerage network; and
- Flooding in most areas within the city during rains;

The public health implications of these conditions cannot be overstated. Consider the case of streets with no, or malfunctioning, street lights. This problem can lead to an increase in the level of traffic accidents involving motorists as well as pedestrians. In addition, the lack of lighting can also negatively impact people's psychological health and wellbeing. Most people who can indulge in physical activity such as walking, cycling and jogging only during the cool hours of the night are unlikely to do so without street lights. Thus, to the extent that physical activities have health benefits, by discouraging such activities the absence of lighting must therefore be seen as antithetical to good health. In addition, darkness is typically linked to social vice. Whether rooted in fact or perception, this association has far-reaching psychological implications, and contributes to social isolation for members of vulnerable groups such as women and the elderly. A number of empirical studies have actually supported this assertion. One such study that comes to mind was conducted in Wales with the support of the Association of Public Health Observatories (see Green, 2009). The study stated that prominent among the health and wellbeing implications of unlit streets are (para. 3):

> an increase in accidents and injuries, possible increase in depression from longer time in darkness and not being able to go out through community safety fears, and possible increased associated costs to primary and secondary health care and social services.

The absence of sufficient street-lights in Lagos is only partially a problem of lack of maintenance and upkeep. Frequently, the problem arises from complete blackouts due to power outages. The health consequences of such outages dwarf those associated with inadequate, or absence of, street lighting. Power outages mean among other things that perishable food cannot be refrigerated; medications and other medical supplies or equipment requiring electric energy or electrically regulated temperatures become dysfunctional or unusable. It also means people must resort to primitive energy sources such as kerosene that are likely to significantly contribute to environmental pollution.

From the aforementioned case, it is clear that deterioration in physical, and especially hygiene and sanitation conditions has direct health consequences. In fact, there is a growing body of works suggesting a direct link between sanitation conditions and most childhood diseases in cities in developing countries (see e.g., Gandy, 2006). Inadequate access to safe drinking water is the most frequently cited culprit in this regard. Thus, for instance, to better appreciate the health implications of indiscriminately disposing of wastes one needs to simply imagine the impact of such wastes on ground water sources.

The indiscriminate disposal of wastes into open fields or bodies of water constitutes only a small part of the sanitation problematic of the megacity of Lagos. Other problems include poor waste disposal habits on the part of the city's residents, as well as ineffective anti-littering initiatives and the lack of the ability to control individual behaviour on the part of municipal authorities. Consequently, thrash is disposed of on the streets, open spaces, markets, and bus stations. Additionally, drains in homes are known to almost always clog or be completely blocked by solid waste. The Lagos Mainland, more than any other part of the city, is the leading culprit in this connection.

Some efforts have been made to promote understanding of the contents of garbage in Lagos (Adedibu and Okekunle, 1989). By some accounts, almost two per cent (1.5%) of the garbage generated in Lagos Mainland is animal carcasses. These are often disposed of in open refuse dumping grounds or simply dropped along the street. Resulting from this is the pungent ordour that is commonplace in some parts of the city. Of course, concomitant with this are air pollution and diseases of all sorts.

The rapid and unprecedented physical and demographic growth of Lagos coupled with negative trends in the local and international economies spell doom for the city. These trends mean, among other things, that the municipal and federal government witness a severe decline in their revenue generating ability. At the same time, individuals from smaller towns and rural communities were allured by the ever receding mirage of a promise for better living conditions in Lagos. Apart from its direct implication for the city's infrastructure, the inability on the part of the government to undertake capital improvement projects triggered a multitude of sanitation problems.

Prominent in this regard are the following (Adedibu and Okekunle, 1989). First, there are no funds to undertake the genre of systematic studies necessary to accurately project the amount of wastes in both quantitative and qualitative terms that is expected during any given period. Second, the problem of resource scarcity, especially as the city experienced in the 1980s and 1990s, thwarted any conceivable effort to maintain existing, and/or launch new, waste disposal facilities. Third, severe budgetary shortfalls, coupled with institutional ineptitude, conspire to brew a toxic cocktail of uncoordinated waste management and disposal activities on the part of municipal sanitation and cognate units. Finally, very little has been done to formulate a coherent waste management policy both at the federal and municipal levels. Throw into this mix the undisciplined and reckless waste disposal habits of a significant segment of the city's population, and one is guaranteed a prescription for disaster in the sanitation policy field.

To be sure, these problems have never completely eluded the attention of federal and municipal authorities. In fact, these authorities have attempted, on several occasions to bring some order to the sanitation situation in Lagos. One such attempt involved promulgation by the Federal Government of a Decree in 1985. The avowed purpose of the decree was to regulate environmental sanitation. The decree was promulgated in tandem with calls for state governments to take serious steps to manage and properly dispose of domestic, human and industrial wastes. Another effort on the part of the Federal Government has involved the operation of an annual programme designed to evaluate cities throughout Nigeria on the basis of their cleanliness, and to reward the cleanest one with a cash prize of one million Naira.

## Hygiene and sanitation in Kinshasa, Congo (DR)

Kinshasa is the only city in Africa that was established by Belgian colonial authorities. Originally designed in the 1960s for a population of 400,000, the city currently has more than eight and a half million (8.6 million) inhabitants (World Bank, 2008). Geographically, the city sits on a flat plain extending to hilly areas in the background. It is swampy in some areas and sits on a foundation of unstable soil in others. In terms of water and sanitation, the city suffers from the same types of problems experienced by human settlements throughout the continent. However, it is worth noting that the problems are generally at a more heightened level in Kinshasa. According to the World Bank (2008), only 18 per cent of the population of this megacity has onsite water; 54 per cent depends on public standpipes, while 38 per cent, almost all of whom are poor, have no access to piped water at all. Only 300,000 cubic meter of the water supplied to the city is treated. This leaves a shortfall of treated water of no less than 400 cubic meters daily.

The human waste disposal system in Kinshasa includes a septic tank in the case of upper-income households. As for low-income household, the system of choice usually includes a pit latrine with superstructures built of non-durable material such as jute bags, scrap metal and palm leaves. Most of these units last for hardly more than 2 to 3 months. On the whole, the city has no sewer systems, and few storm water drainage systems. Where these exist, they serve as de facto sewerage systems through illegal connection of toilet drains. There is a complete absence of a central sewerage system. The latrine evacuating system in place is of the manual genre and only being experimented at this time. The evacuation of fecal sludge in this system is undertaken by way of a hand-operated pump.

The scarcity of safe drinking water is also another public health problem menacing human settlements in the Democratic Republic of Congo. However, it would be grossly erroneous to attribute this problem to a shortage of water sources. In fact, an overwhelming majority (91%) of the sources are unprotected. To be sure, the Congolese territory is richly endowed with water sources. Thus the problem results from ineffective mechanism for the production, transportation and delivery of water from its source to human settlements. According to an IMF Poverty Reduction Strategy Paper for the country, only 22 per cent of the country's urban population has access to safe drinking water (IMF, 2006). Those with access tend to be unevenly spread across the country.

As already observed, water and sanitation conditions in the West and Central Africa sub-region tend to leave much to be desired. However, the situation in Kinshasa in particular and the Congo Democratic Republic in general needs to be evaluated in the context of recent events in that country. The country is emerging from a series of internal strives and violent conflicts. The consequences have included serious damages to the country's water and sanitation infrastructure. The fact that the country, like others in the region, have a history of institutional ineptitude, has only served to aggravate the situation.

The situation has caught the attention not only of the national leadership but the international development community. At the national level, the Congolese leadership has embarked on efforts to enact new water and sanitation policies and revise existing ones. National authorities have also partnered with international entities to accelerate efforts geared towards achieving the Millennium Development Goals in water and sanitation. However, most of the more impactful efforts have occurred at the international level. Particularly noteworthy in this regard are the collaborative initiatives of the United Nations Children's Fund (UNICEF) and the World Health Organization (WHO). Together, these two entities have helped to significantly increase sanitation coverage and access to safe water in Kinshasa and the rest of Congo (DR) (see UNICEF/WHO, 2006). The UNICEF Water and Hygiene Annual Report for 2006 credited these efforts with facilitating access to improved water and sanitation services for 500,000 inhabitants of Congo (DR) (UNICEF, 2006: 20). In addition, they have led sectoral monitoring efforts through the Joint Monitoring Programme (JMP). Furthermore, and particularly important for the purpose of the discussion in this chapter, are UNICEF-led initiatives to develop preliminary codes and guidelines that feed into new sanitation policies. One upshot of initiatives on this front has been the establishment of new or modified national guidelines on water hygiene and sanitation (WASH) in Congolese schools.

International health entities have also been preoccupied with efforts to deal with the consequences of past institutional failures in the country's hygiene and sanitation sector. UNICEF's efforts during the 2006 cholera and diarrhea outbreaks that wreaked havoc in Congo (DR) and other countries in the sub-region is a case in point. The organization provided support to community and household water chlorination programmes, water trucking, hygiene and sanitation promotion as well as technical assistance training and supplies for treatment centers (UNICEF, 2006: 20).

**Conclusion**

This chapter has focused on West and Central Africa, a sub-region of the African continent as delineated by UNICEF and WHO. The sub-region is reputed for having some of the worst sanitation conditions in the world today. In addition, despite being richly endowed with sources of water, including rivers, fresh water lakes and aquifers, the sub-region sits at the bottom of the ladder for access to improved water. In fact, as discussed in this chapter, the sub-region is not on track to attain the water and sanitation target of the Millennium Development Goals (MDGs). However, it is important to note that the poor water and sanitation conditions of the region predated the establishment of the MDGs. A significant proportion of the problems is attributable to colonial human settlement policies. These policies were systematically biased against areas inhabited by Africans as they sought to attend exclusively to the sanitation and related needs of European enclaves. With the passage of time and rapid population growth, but no commensurate investment in water and sanitation infrastructure, the situation grew worse. Thus the current situation is a product of several years of inattentiveness to the sanitation infrastructure of human settlements in the sub-region. If there is anything positive worth mentioning with respect to the water and sanitation situation in the region, it is that these gloomy statistics have caught the attention of authorities at the national and international levels.

# Chapter 7

# Hygiene and Sanitation in the Eastern and Southern Africa Region

## Introduction

This chapter focuses on hygiene and sanitation conditions in the Eastern and Southern Africa region. It is particularly concerned with the nature of the region's hygiene and sanitation problems as well as the initiatives that have been summoned to resolve them. Also of essence are government institutions with major responsibilities in the water and sanitation policy field. Finally, it sheds light on major constraints to efforts to facilitate access to improved water and sanitation in the region. The chapter employs the definition of 'access to improved water and sanitation' proffered by the World Health Organization (WHO) and the United Nations Children's Fund (UNICEF). Thus, access is viewed as the proportion of a country's or city's population that uses improved sanitation facilities. The WHO/UNICEF's definition of improved sanitation includes any system that is capable of systematically separating human excreta from human contact. The Joint Monitoring Programme (JMP) of WHO/UNICEF further proposes a classification scheme that permits the international comparison of these systems. The scheme contains two major categories, namely 'improved' and 'unimproved' sanitation facilities. The improved sanitation systems or facilities include three types. The first is flush or pour flush, which is typically linked to piped sewer, septic tank, or pit latrine. The second type is the ventilated improved pit latrine (VIP). The third is the pit latrine with slab. Finally, there is the composting toilet. The unimproved sanitation system includes five different but overlapping types, viz., flush or pour flush to a different location, pit latrine without slab or open pit, the bucket toilet, the hanging toilet or hanging latrine, and no facilities at all, which implies open defecation. Improved water includes all potable water systems. Access to improved water is typically facilitated by making such water available within convenient reach of users.

The water and sanitation target of the Millennium Development Goals (MDGs) is used as a basis for making any evaluative comments in the chapter. The chapter begins by providing background information on the Eastern and Southern Africa region. Then, it highlights the sanitation conditions in this region. Two subsequent sections respectively identify major constraints to, and the institutional frameworks for promoting, hygiene and sanitation in the region. Following this is a survey of water and sanitation conditions in select major cities in the region. This is followed by a discussion of opportunities and barriers to improved water and sanitation initiatives in the region.

## The Eastern and Southern Africa region

The Eastern and Southern Africa Region as delineated by the United Nations Children's Fund (UNICEF) contains 21 sovereign countries.

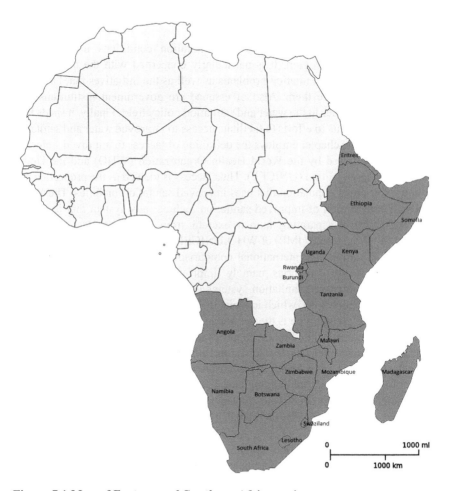

**Figure 7.1 Map of Eastern and Southern Africa region**

*Source*: Author's rendition based on blank map from the 'freely-licensed educational media content' world wide website, Wikimedia Commons at http://commons.wikimedia.rg/wiki/category:blank_maps_of_Africa.

These countries are listed on Table 7.1 and shown on Figure 7.1. As the map (Figure 7.1) shows, the countries differ in geographic size. They range from geographically large countries such as South Africa, Ethiopia and Angola to small ones such as Lesotho, Swaziland, Burundi and Rwanda. The countries also vary significantly in terms of their population size. For instance, as Table 7.1 shows, while Seychelles contained just over 84,000, Ethiopia had more than 80 million inhabitants in 2010 (WHO/UNICEF, 2010).

At the same time, the countries share many attributes in common. Like their other African peers, the countries are erstwhile colonies of one or another European power. Two exceptions, Ethiopia and Eritrea, are worth noting. Yet, it is necessary to note that despite what official records may say, these two countries experienced what for all practical purposes amounts to colonization by the Italians at one point and the British at another. The British controlled the Lion's share of the region as colonial powers. Up until the conclusion of World War I, the Germans controlled Tanganyika (present-day, Tanzania), Burundi, Rwanda, and Namibia. Once the War ended (circa, 1916), the League of Nations took control of all erstwhile German colonies and made them Trust Territories. Under this arrangement, Burundi and Rwanda were placed under the colonial auspices of France. South Africa was charged with overseeing the affairs of Namibia, while Britain was charged with the control of Tanzania. From the onset of the colonial era, France had taken control of the Comoros, Madagascar, and Seychelles. On its part, Britain controlled Zimbabwe (formerly, Southern Rhodesia), Malawi (at the time, Northern Rhodesia), Uganda, Kenya, South Africa, Swaziland, Lesotho, and Botswana. Portugal had two colonies, namely Mozambique and Angola in the region. A common thread that ran through the governance philosophies of these disparate colonial powers is racial residential segregation. Racial residential segregation had far-reaching implications for the distribution of hygiene and sanitation facilities in human settlements throughout the continent. As argued in this book, the hygiene and sanitation problematic in Africa today is an embodiment and reflection of colonial urban planning philosophy.

Table 7.1 demonstrates without equivocation that countries in the region have a long way to go to meet the hygiene-and-sanitation-related targets of the Millennium Development Goals (MDGs). A more noteworthy aspect of the table is the revelation that, unhygienic practices such as open defecation remain rampant in the sub-region. In this regard, Eritrea lays claim to a dubious record. It is the country with the highest incidence of open defecation in urban areas. As much as 41 per cent of the urban population in this country practices open defecation. The situation is worse in rural areas. In rural Eritrea, for instance, almost everyone (96%) practices open defecation. Closely behind Eritrea are Namibia and Ethiopia, where, respectively 71 per cent and 73 per cent of the rural population practices open defecation. Table 7.1 also suggests that the hygiene and sanitation situation in the sub-region is not completely bleak. A large proportion of the urban population in some countries in the region, including Seychelles (97%), Angola (86%), and South Africa (84%), has access to improved sanitation facilities.

Table 7.1 Sanitation conditions in the Eastern and Southern Africa region

| Country | Population (X 1,000) | Urban (%) | | | | Rural (%) | | | |
|---|---|---|---|---|---|---|---|---|---|
| | | Improved | Shared | Unimproved | Open defecation | Improved | Shared | Unimproved | Open defecation |
| Angola | | 86 | – | 13 | 1 | 18 | – | 29 | 53 |
| Botswana | 1,921 | 74 | 7 | 18 | 1 | 39 | 11 | 12 | 38 |
| Burundi | 8,074 | 49 | 22 | 27 | 2 | 46 | 4 | 49 | 1 |
| Comoros | 661 | 50 | 3 | 46 | 1 | 30 | 2 | 68 | 0 |
| Eritrea | 4,927 | 52 | – | 7 | 41 | 4 | – | 0 | 96 |
| Ethiopia | 80,713 | 29 | 34 | 29 | 8 | 8 | 2 | 19 | 71 |
| Kenya | 38,765 | 27 | 51 | 20 | 2 | 32 | 18 | 32 | 18 |
| Lesotho | 2,049 | 40 | 35 | 17 | 8 | 25 | 3 | 21 | 51 |
| Madagascar | 19,111 | 15 | 28 | 39 | 18 | 10 | 17 | 35 | 38 |
| Malawi | 14,846 | 51 | 42 | 5 | 2 | 57 | 24 | 8 | 11 |
| Mozambique | 22,383 | 38 | 7 | 41 | 14 | 4 | 1 | 36 | 59 |
| Namibia | 2,130 | 60 | 17 | 5 | 18 | 17 | 4 | 6 | 73 |
| Rwanda | 9,721 | 50 | 18 | 31 | 1 | 55 | 6 | 36 | 3 |
| Seychelles | 0.892 | 97 | – | 2 | 1 | – | – | – | – |
| Somalia | 8,926 | 52 | 30 | 15 | 3 | 6 | 6 | 5 | 83 |
| South Africa | 49,668 | 84 | 10 | 4 | 2 | 65 | 9 | 9 | 17 |
| Swaziland | 1,168 | 61 | 32 | 5 | 2 | 53 | 20 | 6 | 21 |
| Tanzania | 42,484 | 32 | 30 | 36 | 2 | 21 | 21 | 41 | 17 |
| Uganda | 31,657 | 38 | 56 | 4 | 2 | 49 | 22 | 18 | 11 |
| Zambia | 12,620 | 59 | 22 | 17 | 2 | 43 | 9 | 22 | 26 |
| Zimbabwe | 12,463 | 56 | 40 | 2 | 2 | 37 | 15 | 9 | 39 |

Source: Based on data from WHO/UNICEF (2010).

## Trends in sanitation coverage in the region

The East and Southern Africa region has made modest progress in sanitation during the last two decades. Table 7.2 shows the region's gains vis-à-vis those of other regions on the continent between 1990 and 2006. The table contains data on two extreme cases, namely 'improved sanitation facilities' and 'open defecation.' Modest progress was registered in both cases throughout the continent. In Eastern Africa, the proportion of the population with access to improved sanitation facilities increased from 25 to 29 per cent between 1990 and 2006. Thus, far less than half of the population in this sub-region has access to improved sanitation facilities. It is informative to evaluate the region's sanitation situation within its broader continental context. In this regard, it is worth noting that the region's sanitation situation is better than that of West Africa. However, it compares unfavourably to what obtains on average throughout the African continent. The situation is significantly better in the Southern Africa sub-region. Here, more than half of the population has access to improved sanitation facilities. However, the sub-region's gains on this score were also modest. In this connection, the proportion of its population with access to improved sanitation facilities increased from 52 to 57 per cent. Improvements in the area of open defecation were better in both the Southern and Eastern Africa sub-regions. In the Eastern Africa sub-region, the proportion of the population practicing open defecation dropped by more than ten per cent from 44 per cent in 1990 to 33 per cent in 2006. In the Southern Africa sub-region, the decrease in the percentage practicing open defecation was from 16 to 13 per cent between 1990 and 2006.

**Table 7.2 Progress in sanitation in Africa, 1990–2006**

| Region | Improved Facilities (% of Population) | | Open Defecation (% of Population) | |
|---|---|---|---|---|
| | 1990 | 2006 | 1990 | 2006 |
| Eastern Africa | 25 | 29 | 44 | 33 |
| Southern Africa | 52 | 57 | 16 | 13 |
| West Africa | 21 | 25 | 36 | 29 |
| North Africa | 57 | 68 | 20 | 11 |
| All Africa | 33 | 38 | 33 | 24 |

*Source*: Based on data from WHO/UNICEF (2008).

**Table 7.3 Access to improved sources of water in East and Southern Africa, 2008**

| Country | Surface area (Km²) | Percent urban pop. | Improved water coverage (%) | | |
|---|---|---|---|---|---|
| | | | Urban | Rural | Total |
| Angola | 1,246,700 | 59 | 60 | 38 | 50 |
| Botswana | 581,730 | 61 | 99 | 90 | 95 |
| Burundi | 27,830 | 11 | 83 | 71 | 72 |
| Comoros | 2,235 | 28 | 91 | 97 | 95 |
| Eritrea | 117,600 | 22 | 74 | 57 | 61 |
| Ethiopia | 1,104,300 | 17 | 98 | 26 | 38 |
| Kenya | 580 | 22 | 83 | 52 | 59 |
| Lesotho | 30,355 | 27 | 97 | 81 | 85 |
| Madagascar | 587,041 | 30 | 71 | 29 | 41 |
| Malawi | 118,484 | 20 | 95 | 77 | 80 |
| Mozambique | 799,380 | 38 | 77 | 29 | 47 |
| Namibia | 824,292 | 38 | 99 | 88 | 92 |
| Rwanda | 26,338 | 19 | 77 | 62 | 65 |
| Seychelles | 455 | 55 | 100 | – | – |
| Somalia | 637,657 | 37 | 67 | 9 | 30 |
| South Africa | 1,219,090 | 62 | 99 | 65 | 77 |
| Swaziland | 17,364 | 21 | 92 | 61 | 69 |
| Tanzania | 947,300 | 26 | 80 | 45 | 54 |
| Uganda | 241,038 | 13 | 91 | 64 | 67 |
| Zambia | 752,618 | 36 | 87 | 46 | 60 |
| Zimbabwe | 390,757 | 38 | 99 | 72 | 82 |

*Source*: Compiled based on data from the US CIA Factbook: https://www.cia.gov/library/publications/the-world-factbook/wfbExt/region_afr.html.

It helps to disaggregate the statistics on the progress in sanitation that has been registered throughout the entire region since the 1990s. One vital piece of information that can be unveiled through this exercise is that most of the gains in sanitation conditions registered were for urban areas. On their own, the statistics tend to disguise or understate the severity of the region's sanitation problems. This is especially true given that as many as 24 million people in the region still practice open defecation (WHO/UNICEF, 2008). The national figures on open defecation are also worthy of note. South Africa boasts the most extensive sewerage coverage as well as the most impressive inventory of other sanitation infrastructure in the region. Yet, almost 20 million (19.7 million) of its residents practiced open defecation in 2006. In Swaziland, one of the smallest countries in the region, more than half a million (0.6 million) people indulged in this practice that same year.

In general, the pace at which progress in hygiene and sanitation has historically been made in the region is chronically sluggish. The following fact serves to bolster this assertion. More than three decades ago, the UN-General Assembly declared 1980–1990 the Water and Sanitation Decade. This declaration was intended to draw attention to the magnitude of the water and sanitation problem throughout the world. More importantly, it was meant to ensure that everyone had access to improved water and sanitation. At the end of said decade in 1990, the efforts had failed to register any significant success. The gains made during that decade fell significantly below the ten per cent increase realized prior to the Declaration. Were progress in water and sanitation to continue at this pace, it would take more than a century, and over 30 billion dollars (US) to achieve total sanitation in the region (p. 7).

As Table 7.3 shows, the Eastern and Southern Africa region has a better record on access to improved sources of water than on improved sanitation. This is understandable given that the region is blessed with vast sources of fresh water. It boasts the largest fresh water lakes (e.g., Lake Victoria/Nyansa, and Lake Tanganyika), and is the source of the longest river in the world, namely River Nile.

## Institutional frameworks

A common feature of governments in Africa is their sheer size. In other words, African governments are typically outsized or bloated. One manifestation of this phenomenon is the presence of an excessive number of government institutions operating in any given policy field. The World Bank/International Monetary Fund (IMF)-initiated structural adjustment programmes (SAP) dating back to the 1980s have succeeded in curtailing the size of bureaucracies on the continent. However, the programmes have been more effective in slashing the public labour force than in reducing the number of public sector institutional actors. In many cases, the net number of government institutions remained virtually intact or actually increased. It is easy to follow this line of reasoning once one understands that the SAPs led to the emergence of previously unknown ministerial bodies in Africa. Examples include ministries with functions such as 'administrative reforms,' 'government decentralization' that can be found in almost every country on the continent today.

It is common to find an unwarranted number of government institutions in charge of a single substantive policy. This often leads to inefficiency and ineffectiveness especially at the policy implementation level. The notions that African bureaucracies are bloated, and that this is a leading cause of Africa's socio-economic failures, have not gone unchallenged. For instance, Goldsmith (1999) contended that African bureaucracies are not atypical. In fact, they are, he argued, relatively smaller than those of other developing regions such as Asia. He employed the case of Botswana, a country with a relatively large public sector, to challenge the hypothesis of large size as a cause of socio-economic failure. Yet, it bears noting that Goldsmith's is a minority viewpoint. The view that African bureaucracies are bloated is widespread. This view was at the root of the World Bank/IMF recommendation that African governments trim the excess fat in their bureaucracies as part of SAPs. In fact, the dictum that 'government is best that governs least' richly laces most of the administrative reform recommendations often made to African governments (see e.g., Kyambalesa, 2004).

Countries in the Eastern and Southern Africa region typify the 'bloated bureaucracy syndrome.' This assertion appears most apropos with respect to the water and sanitation sector. It is commonplace, as shown on Table 7.4, to find multiple ministerial bodies simultaneously formulating, implementing, monitoring and evaluating water supply and sanitation policies. Consider the case of Kenya. At least five ministerial bodies have some responsibility in the water and sanitation policy field. These bodies include the Ministry of Water and Irrigation, the Ministry of Public Health and Sanitation, the Ministry for Nairobi Metropolitan Development, the Ministry of Development of Northern Kenya and other Arid Lands, and the Ministry of Public Works. Two of these ministries, the Ministry of Public Health and Sanitation, and the Ministry of Water and Irrigation, have vision and mission statements that are indistinguishable. The mission statement of the Ministry of Public Health and Sanitation reads as follows (Government of Kenya, Online):

> The Ministry of Public Health and Sanitation has as its fundamental goal and purpose as conserving, managing and protecting water resources for socio-economic development.

On its part, the Ministry of Water and Irrigation articulates its mission as follows (Ibid):

> Integrated water resources management and development through stakeholder participation to ensure availability and accessibility to enhance national development.

## Table 7.4 Government ministries in water and sanitation, East and Central Africa region

| Country | Ministries with Responsibility in the Water and Sanitation Sector |
|---------|---------------------------------------------------------------------|
| Angola | 1) Ministry of Energy & Water; 2) Ministry of Urban Affairs & Construction; 3) Ministry of Health. |
| Botswana | 1) Ministry of Health; 2) Ministry of Minerals, Energy & Water Resources; 3) Ministry of Lands. |
| Burundi | 1) Ministry of Public Health & Fight Against AIDS; 2) Ministry of Planning & Communal Development; 3) Ministry of Energy & Mines. |
| Comoros | 1) Ministry of Land, Urbanism & Housing; 2) Ministry of Health, Solidarity, Social Cohesion & Gender Promotion. |
| Eritrea | 1) Ministry of Health; 2) Ministry of Land, Water & Environment; 3) Ministry of Public Works. |
| Ethiopia | 1) Ministry of Health; 2) Ministry of Urban Development; 3) Ministry of Water & Energy. |
| Kenya | 1) Ministry of Public Health & Sanitation; 2) Ministry of Water & Irrigation; 3) Ministry for Nairobi Metropolitan Development; Ministry for Development of Northern Kenya & Other Arid Lands. |
| Lesotho | 1) Ministry of Health & Social Welfare; 2) Ministry of Public Works & Transport. |
| Madagascar | 1) Ministry of Public Health; 2) Ministry of Public Works & Meteorology; 3) Ministry of Water. |
| Malawi | 1) Ministry of Agriculture, Irrigation & Water; 2) Ministry of Health; 3) Ministry of Land, Housing & Urban Development. |
| Mauritius | 1) Ministry of Health & Quality of Life; 2) Ministry of Housing & Lands; 3) Ministry of Public Infrastructure & Development. |
| Mozambique | 1) Ministry of Health; 2) Ministry of Public Works. |
| Namibia | 1) Ministry of Agriculture, Water & Forestry; 2) Ministry of Health & Social Welfare; 3) Ministry of Regional & Local Government & Housing & Rural Dev. |
| Rwanda | 1) Ministry of Health; 2) Ministry of Infrastructure; 3) Ministry of Local Government, Good Governance, Community Development & Social Affairs. |
| Seychelles | 1) Ministry of Health; 2) Ministry of Lands & Housing. |
| Somalia | 1) Ministry of Health & Human Services; 2) Ministry of Mineral Resources, Water, Energy & Petroleum; 3) Ministry of Public Works & Reconstruction. |
| South Africa | 1) Ministry of Human Settlements; 2) Ministry of Health; 3) Ministry of Water & Environmental Affairs. |
| Swaziland | 1) Ministry of Health; 2) Ministry of Local Government & Housing; 3) Ministry of Public Works & Transport. |
| Tanzania | 1) Ministry of Health & Social Welfare; 2) Ministry of Water; 3) Ministry of Lands & Human Settlements; 4) Ministry of Infrastructure Development. |
| Uganda | 1) Ministry of Lands, Housing & Urban Development; 2) Ministry of Health; Ministry of Water & Environment. |
| Zambia | 1) Ministry of Health; 2) Ministry of Lands, Energy & Water; 3) Ministry of Local Government, Housing, Early Education, & Environment. |
| Zimbabwe | 1) Ministry of Health & Child Welfare; 2) Ministry of Public Works; 3) Ministry of Water Resources Management & Development. |

*Source*: Based on data from National Government Websites & CIA World Factbook (www.cia.gov).

The multiplicity of government institutions operating in a single policy field poses an endless string of problems. At the very least, scarce resources are wasted when there is unnecessary redundancy in efforts to execute any given task. Then, there is the problem of uneven level of service occasioned by difficulties associated with coordinating too many service delivery entities. Above all, too many government agencies often lead to a lack of transparency and accountability. At least one government in the region, namely Botswana is cognizant of these problems and is at the forefront of efforts to rectify them. Botswana has an impressive record in undertaking meaningful institutional reforms. From September 2008 to January 2009, the government of that country, with support from the World Bank, carried out institutional reforms in the country's water and sanitation sector (Government of Botswana, Online). The main aim of these reforms was to streamline the sector and ensure separation and responsibility between, a) the delivery of water and sanitation services, and b) the management of water resources.

The foregoing narrative suggests two things. First, several common threads characterize the water and sanitation situation in the Eastern and Southern Africa region. Second, a careful examination of the situation reveals that the problems also tend to differ by country, and even by towns or cities within the same country. To illustrate this point, the following passages examine the state of hygiene and sanitation in select major cities in the region. Of particular interest are Addis Ababa, Ethiopia; Cape Town, South Africa; Dar es Salaam, Tanzania; Harare, Zimbabwe; and Nairobi, Kenya.

*Addis Ababa, Ethiopia*

The population of Addis Ababa, or Addis, as it is fondly known by Ethiopians, was estimated to be about 3 million in 2009 (Hutton, 2007). As part of a landlocked country, the socio-economic problems of Addis Ababa are compounded. The city has access to only one river, the Akaki River. Climatically, the city enjoys sub-tropical conditions. At the same time, it constitutes the economic hub of the entire country. Consequently, the city is constantly dealing with problems of pollution. The most significant of these problems are tied to the few industries operating in the city. Prominent in this regard are industrial wastes from tanneries, textiles and food processing plants.

The city has a sanitation master plan. The plan is an updated version of the 1993 master plan. Within the framework of this plan both sewage and faecal sludge are integrated. The city is only minimally served by a central or collective sanitation network. The city's small sewerage network is located in the central area and serves less than three per cent of its population. The network was commissioned in 1981 and presently consists of 30 kilometres of trunk sewer, 90 km of secondary sewers serving about 40,000 people through 1800 connections. Most of the city's sewage is discharged into open drains. It has a number of waste water treatment plants. One of these plants, the Kaiti wastewater plant, has a capacity of 7,600 cubic meters per day (m³/day). Currently, it receives 4,500 m³/day. Another plant, the Kotebe sewer plant receives sludge and discharges it directly into the Awash River. As much as 75 per cent of the households in the city uses pit latrines. Most pit latrines in Addis Ababa are shared by multiple households. There are hardly any public toilets in the city. However, despite the near-absence of public toilets, and sanitation facilities in general, only a very small proportion (5 per cent) of the city's residents resorts to open defecation. One factor accounting for this anomaly is the indigenous ethos of Ethiopia, which frowns on open defecation or indiscreet disposal of human waste.

## Cape Town, South Africa

National Census records by Statistics South Africa (SSA, 2007) contain vital information on hygiene and sanitation conditions in cities and towns throughout South Africa. According to one of the most recent of these records Cape Town had a population of 3.7 million in 2007 (SSA, 2007). The sanitation conditions of this city are superior to those of other cities in sub-Saharan Africa in general and the Eastern and Southern Africa region in particular. This is mainly, although not exclusively, a function of two factors. First, the city was initially developed as a settler city in a settler colony. Therefore, it was intended as an exclusive European enclave. Secondly, South Africa of which the city is a part enjoys a level of socio-economic development that is superior to those of its regional and continental peers. On the negative side, Cape Town, like other coastal cities, tends to suffer from problems such as flooding. Cape Town also boasts more manufacturing and industrial activities than most African cities. Consequently, it wrestles with pollution problems that are unknown or only little-known elsewhere in the region. These problems include, but are not limited to pollutants from food processing, oil refining, chemicals, plastics and cement manufacturing.

Water resources in Cape Town include dams, especially the Kleinplass Dam on the Eerste River and a number of ground sources. Most of the households (91 per cent) in the city have on-plot piped water, while 8 per cent depends on piped water from public standpipes. Only one per cent of the population is without access to piped water. Sanitation access is equally generous in Cape Town. In fact, as is the case with other basic needs, the level of accessibility to sanitation facilities is far above what obtains in most cities throughout the region. Only six per cent of the population is considered as having inadequate sanitation based on the World Bank/United Nations definition. Ninety-one per cent of households in the city have flush toilets. More noteworthy is the fact that these toilets are connected to an extensive city-wide sewerage system. The sewerage system covers most of the Cape Town Metropolitan area. Septic tanks, which constitute the norm in most cities in the Eastern and Southern Africa region, are uncommon in Cape Town. Only two per cent of the households in the city have flush toilets that are connected to septic tanks. However, an unusually large proportion (7 per cent) of the population uses bucket toilets systems or latrines.

Another area in which Cape Town commands superiority over cities in other countries in the region has to do with sanitation in low-income districts. It can be stated without equivocation that few if any cities in Africa have better sanitation services in their informal and poor districts than Cape Town. Cape Town's poor and/or low-income districts boast government-provided and maintained public toilets. The toilets are of various technological specifications and standards. However, on the average, the services they provide are the equivalence of less than one latrine per household. Garbage collection, a relatively rare service in most cities throughout the Eastern and Southern Africa region, is provided on a regular basis in Cape Town. Open defecation is a rarity. Sewerage treatment in Cape Town is comparable to those of other cities in the developed world. The city has 22 waste water treatment plants. Of these, 21 are owned and operated by municipal authorities, while one is privately-owned and operated.

*Dar es Salaam, Tanzania*

As Brinkhoff (2010) noted, Dar es Salaam, Tanzania's most populated city has a population of a little more than 3 million (3.1 million). It is Africa's third fastest growing city after Bamako and Lagos. Dar es Salaam is a coastal city characterized by swamps in some areas and steep slopes in others. Hygiene and sanitation authorities in Dar es Salaam have a number of problems to worry about. Prominent in this regard are pollutants originating from a number of the city's industrial and manufacturing activities, including food processing, textiles, tanneries, fertilizers and petroleum refining. As for water, the Pangani River, which also goes by the name River Ruvu, constitutes an important source. The river is important not only as a source of potable water, but also a major source of hydroelectric energy in Tanzania. It has a production capacity that is capable of supplying water to the city's current population. However, there are some problems with transmission, storage capacity and treatment quality.

Another river, the Msimbazi River, dissects the City of Dar es Salaam into almost two equal parts to the North and South. A few facts about the river are worth mentioning here particularly because of their implications for hygiene and sanitation in that city. As Lugalla (1997) has stated, the river constitutes a viable, and in some cases, the only, source of drinking water for families without access to pipe borne water. However, because the river also serves as a receptacle for industrial waste in the city, especially the industries located along Pugu Road, it constitutes a direct threat to the health of the poor in the area. In fact, the entire Msimbazi River basin is eminently dangerous in this regard. This is particularly because further west, and precisely in the Vingunguti area, the basin serves as home to the biggest solid waste dump in Dar es Salaam.

Its salubrious conditions notwithstanding, the Msimbazi River Basin serves as the home for many urban poor in Dar es Salaam. Lugalla characterizes the area as comprising housing units of simple and impermanent building materials such as mud, sticks, recycled metal and thatched grass roofs. The shoddy improvised housing units are poorly ventilated, and in most cases, not ventilated at all. Additionally, density levels in the area are generally very high, with very little room for outdoor recreation, or the proper disposal of domestic waste. Concomitant with the high density is the problem of overcrowding. It is not uncommon for different families to live under the same roof, and share basic facilities. According to one study, "more than four people may live, cook, eat and sleep in one room" (Lugalla, 1997: 22).

Other revelations of the afore-cited study with implications for public health include the following. Most households (71%) in the area are not officially connected to the city's electricity grid. This is partially due to the expensive, tedious and cumbersome process associated with officially obtaining electricity connection in the city. Consequently, residents resort to illegal power connections, which are in and of themselves serious health hazards. As stated earlier, pipe borne water is almost non-existent in the low-income, and especially informal settlements. This is especially true of the Kinondoni-Hananasif and Vingunguti settlements. Here, as in similar settlements throughout Dar es Salaam, only a small proportion (9.4%) of the households has flush toilets, while the majority depends on pit latrines for the disposal of human excreta (Ibid, 23). Paradoxically, pit latrines also double as garbage pits (Ibid). Also worth noting is the fact that pit latrines tend to be shallow because of the city's high water table. In addition, the latrines are typically located within close proximity to drinking water wells. The health implications of this are obvious and need not be regurgitated here.

The city's drainage system, wherever this exists, is generally of sub-standard quality. In fact, most areas within the city have no drainage system for storm and surface water at all. Also, waste pits are a rarity. Consequently, a significant number of households tends to discard domestic wastes on the streets. Garbage collection is rare, irregular or non-existent in some cases. Consequently, as Lugalla (1997: 23) has noted, "garbage is left uncollected and untreated for a longtime." One upshot of the commensurate congestion is the prevalence of communicable diseases such as tuberculosis, influenza, and meningitis.

Sanitation access is similar to what obtains in most cities throughout the region. In this regard, only 10 per cent of the city's population has sewerage connection. According to the World Bank (2003), 20 per cent of city's population—mostly in the upper-income districts—has septic tanks. The rest of the population uses pit latrines. More precisely, as much as 92 per cent of the population uses pit latrines (Allen et al., 2004). These latrines are mainly of the unlined pit variety. A rather unusual and definitely unhealthy method that is typically used to empty pit latrines in the city is known as 'seasonal flushing.' This method entails the use of floodwater to flush the pit latrines' contents into the open. As implied above, this has serious health implications.

The city has a relatively extensive sewer system that runs for as many as 140 kilometres. The system is connected to the ocean outlet or to one of nine decentralized wastewater stabilization ponds. However, it must be noted that informal settlements are not served by this system.

*Harare, Zimbabwe*

Harare was initially developed as a settler colonial city in what was then known as Southern Rhodesia. Currently, the city boasts a population of a little more than 2 million (2.3 million) (Brinkheroff, 2010). The city is located on a high plateau and enjoys a sub-tropical climate. Although it is located on a plateau, it tends to suffer from occasional flooding. The city has extensive industrial activities. This has far-reaching implications for sanitation throughout the city and its proximate environment. For instance, industrial pollution emanating especially from chemicals, textile and cognate production activities are commonplace. Water for the city comes mainly from lakes such as Lakes Chiver and Manyame.

Access to sanitation in Harare is better than in most cities in the region in particular and the African continent in general. Until recently, most inhabitants of Harare, including residents of low-income districts had access to improved sanitation. However, it is important to note that even in its heydays as a settler colonial city, informal districts were locked out of the sanitation grid. In other words, these districts were not served by the sewerage system. Brinkhoff (2010) has reported on the state of Harare's hygiene and sanitation coverage and infrastructure. Currently, the city's sanitation infrastructure is suffering from disrepair and neglect. About 33 per cent of its population uses pour-flush toilets. These toilets discharge into sewers, septic tanks, and open drains. Between 33 and 37 per cent of the city's households have ventilated improved pit (VIP) latrines. However, about 24 to 48 per cent of the households are served by insanitary pit latrines. Between two and 13 per cent of the households have no sanitary facilities at all. Local municipal laws authorize septic tanks only for plots that are at least 2000 square meters.

Sanitation problems in Harare have manifested themselves in several ways. For instance, the 2008/2009 cholera outbreak in Zimbabwe resulted in more deaths in Harare than elsewhere in the country as a whole. Yet, as noted earlier, sanitation conditions and infrastructure in the city remain relatively better than in other major cities throughout the Eastern and Southern Africa region. For instance, the city has an extensive central sewerage system—something that is rare in sub-Saharan Africa in general. Most households in the city's formal settlements or districts, including those within the lower income brackets, are served by the city's central sewer system. Thus, most of the city, accounting for as much as 1.8 million or 80 per cent of the entire Harare Metropolitan area, is hooked to the system. However, it is necessary to note that because of the problem of disrepair mentioned above, the system is largely dysfunctional. Also, it is worthy of note that the system does not extend to informal settlements. This is a legacy of the city's colonial past. During the colonial era, sanitation and hygiene services were restricted exclusively to the European districts. Within this framework, the native settlements were neglected and denied even the most basic of hygiene and sanitation infrastructure and services. These settlements evolved into what has come to be known as informal settlements and low-income districts during the post-colonial era.

Sewage from the City of Harare is routed to two large activated sludge plants. The one, Crowborough, has a capacity of 54,000 cubic meters per day (54,000m³/day). The other, Firle, has a capacity of 144,000 cubic meters per day (144,000m³/day). However, these two plants are not up to the task of handling the volume of wastewater generated by the city. In fact, a lot of its wastewater goes partially, or completely, untreated. The inadequately and partially treated water typically winds up in the Rivers Marimba and Mukuvisi. The rivers in turn drain into Lakes Chivero and Manyame, which are the city's major sources of water. The city also boasts two waste stabilization ponds and an aeration pond. Some of the city's waste water and sludge are applied to pasture.

*Nairobi, Kenya*

With a population of 3.4 million, Nairobi stands out as one of the largest cities in the Eastern and Southern Africa regions. Nairobi enjoys what can be best described as a sub-tropical climate. The city boasts a number of diverse industrial activities. These activities, including chemical processing, textiles, cement manufacturing, and food processing tend to generate pollutants that are not adequately handled. Nairobi is also reputed as a colonial city. Thus, the form of racial residential segregation and the unequal distribution of public infrastructure, especially hygiene and sanitation infrastructure for which colonial cities are well known, constitutes an important element of the city's history. It is an inland city that is located at an altitude of 500 to 1,900 meters above sea level. However, it is flat in the lower segments and characterized by steep slopes in the higher areas. The flat areas of the city tend to be menaced by serious flooding during the rainy season. The city is literally traversed by the River Nairobi and its many tributaries including the Mathare and the Ngong. Other rivers that constitute the major sources of the city's water include the Tana River Basin. Most of the city's potable water originates in this source. However, only the formal residential districts tend to depend on the source for water. The informal districts depend on the heavily polluted River Nairobi, the Mathare and the Ngong. Piped borne water coverage is adequate in the government and institutional office zone, as well as the upper- and middle-income districts but scant in the rest of the city. On the whole, 42 per cent of the households in Nairobi have household piped water supply. In contrast, most people in the informal settlements, including Kibera, depend on street vendours for water.

The United Nations Centre for Human Settlements (UN-Habitat, 2003) has assessed sanitation coverage in Nairobi. An important revelation of the Centre's efforts is the fact that sanitation services and infrastructure tend to be limited to the formal districts, particularly the areas inhabited by upper- and middle-income households. A small proportion (10 per cent) of the households as well as the business and institutional districts are connected to the city's limited central sewer system, while 20 per cent use septic tanks. The remainder depends on latrines. Some of those in the former category have flush toilets, while others have pour-flush toilets.

In the informal districts, that is, where some 60 per cent of the city's population is located, about 24 per cent of the households have latrines. About half of the latrines are of the improved variety while the other half comprises the unimproved and makeshift alternatives. A few public toilets are distributed throughout the city. However, these toilets tend to be overcrowded and poorly maintained. In the low-income and/or informal settlements the scarcity or absence of toilets has led to the adoption of many unconventional methods of human waste disposal. In some cases, plastic bags are used and then indiscriminately disposed of. In as much as 6 per cent of the cases, the people simply resort to open defecation.

As stated earlier, Nairobi has a very limited central sewerage system. By some accounts, this system serves only 10 per cent of the city's population (see e.g., UN-Habitat, 2003). According to some other sources (e.g., Government of Kenya, 2002), the system serves almost half (48 per cent) of the city's population. At any rate, there is no question that only the affluent districts as well as the business and institutional zones are served by the system. In other words, the system does not extend to the low-income and/or informal districts. In these latter areas, latrines are commonplace. These latrines are emptied by tankers. In the informal settlements, the latrines are either poorly constructed or non-existent. Consequently, poor sanitary conditions tend to be the norm in these settlements.

## Barriers and opportunities

As observed above, there is a tendency to attribute every problem that ails Africa to the lack of financial and material resources. This is misleading and portends several negative implications for development initiatives. In fact, such a reductionist view tends to prevent analysts from seeking alternative explanations for the continent's plethora of problems. Certainly, some proportion of the hygiene and sanitation problems plaguing the Eastern and Southern Africa region can be accounted for by the absence of resources. The power of this explanation is reinforced by the fact that the region ranks as one of the most impoverished in the world. However, other factors such as culture, war, drought, and politics may be more portent in explaining the region's low sanitation and water coverage.

*Culture*

Most of what is required to improve hygiene and sanitation conditions anywhere has to do with behaviour modification. In other words, simply modifying people's hygiene behaviour holds enormous promise for efforts to address many sanitation questions. The implied link between culture and sanitation becomes more obvious once one appreciates the fact that many behavioural patterns are a function of culture. This culture may be of the indigenous or received variety. Thus, any meaningful attempt to institute behaviour modification initiatives as a means of improving sanitation conditions in the region must be attentive to both variants of culture.

A report on a training workshop on 'community-led total sanitation' that took place in Zambia from 14 to 18 July 2008 contains very insightful information in this connection (see PZ/RESA, 2008). The report noted the role of indigenous culture and beliefs in derailing sanitation initiatives in the region. A word on the 'community-led total sanitation' (CLTS) sanitation strategy is necessary before delving any further into the cultural dimensions of sanitation. The strategy is not novel. In fact, its history in the region dates back to the late-1990s. It has been defined as

> an approach which facilitates a process of empowering local communities to
> stop open defecation and to build and use latrines without the support of any
> external hardware (PZ/RESA, 2008: 8).

The approach is different from others that have been tried in the past. This is especially because it recognizes the real and potential role of tradition and culture in encouraging or discouraging unhygienic and salubrious behaviour.

Indigenous culture and beliefs have been known to lead to failures in sanitation and hygiene initiatives in the sub-Saharan region as a whole and the Eastern and Southern Africa region in particular (PZ/RESA, 2008). For instance, there are indigenous beliefs that promote the notion that pregnant women can suffer a miscarriage if they shared sanitation facilities such as latrines with men. In a similar light, some indigenous beliefs in the region hold that a man's testicles would swell if he shared sanitation facilities with women. The view of elders and children sharing hygiene and sanitation facilities as a taboo is also harboured by some of the indigenous belief systems within the region. Furthermore, some indigenous groups in the region believe that the use of closed systems such as latrines for defecation constitutes a selfish act on the part of humans. Within the context of this belief system, open defecation is endorsed as a means of providing food to pigs and other creatures that feed on human wastes. While elements of these and other indigenous beliefs may be logical, efforts to promote proper hygiene and sanitation must first and foremost focus on ensuring the separation of human wastes from human beings. Consequently, certain cultural practices and beliefs must be discouraged in order to achieve this goal.

However, there is the danger of indiscriminately discarding all cultural practices and beliefs in the name of modernization. Those charged with the responsibility for promoting proper hygiene and sanitation are beseeched to eschew this temptation. Rather, they must appreciate some indigenous knowledge and concomitant practices as assets in efforts to promote sustainable sanitation initiatives. At least one example is in order. Most African cultures see all bodies of water, including rivers, lakes, and the sea as sacred. In fact, bodies of water are seen not only as God's gift to humans and all earthly creatures but also God's abode. Based on African indigenous ethos, humans can therefore not own any body of water. They are also not at liberty to treat any water source as they please. More importantly for the purpose of the present discussion, humans are forbidden from desecrating, especially through defecation, any and all bodies of water.

Such thinking that deified bodies of water was long a casualty of modernization. Agents of modernization derided Africans for harbouring beliefs that viewed bodies of water as anything but natural resources, which humans could treat as they saw fit. Although environmental awareness has led to serious re-thinking about how natural resources, including water ought to be treated, there has been very little, if any acknowledgement of the foresightedness of African indigenous knowledge in this regard. Yet, it may take enlisting this knowledge and re-instituting the concomitant beliefs for efforts to discourage defecation in lakes, rivers and other bodies of water to succeed.

*War*

Another prominent factor that has served as a barrier to developing or improving access to, improved water and sanitation facilities in the region is war. At least five countries, including Angola, Ethiopia, Eritrea, Mozambique and Uganda, in the region have been victimized by war. War has inevitable consequences for water supply and sanitation. Consider the case of Angola. The country suffered a prolonged war for 27 years. This war, which ended less than a decade ago, was extremely costly not only in terms of human life. Rather, it also resulted in irreversible damage to the country's water supply and sanitation systems. In addition, the war displaced many people, especially from the countryside. As one report by the United Nations Children's Fund (UNICEF) noted, most of the displaced people ended up in towns and peri-urban areas (UNICEF, 2008). Consequently, the fragile water and sanitation systems of these areas are overtaxed. The report further observed that most foreign assistance projects, including those of UNICEF itself, tend to be dedicated to improving access to potable water. This means, among other things, that hygiene and sanitation are often neglected. Eritrea and Ethiopia, two of the most impoverished countries in the region were involved in a two-year border war (1998–2000). Specific statistics on the sanitation-related damage inflicted by the war are unavailable. However, UNICEF (2008) reported that the war internally displaced at least 1.2 million. If nothing else, this displacement resulted in straining not only the impoverished countries' healthcare system but also their precarious water and sanitation infrastructure.

Mozambique witnessed a bloody civil war that pitted the Front for Liberation of Mozambique (FRELIMO) against the Mozambique Resistance Movement (RENAMO) from 1977 to 1992. The war claimed almost a million lives and permanently maimed hundreds of thousands more. Although it is about two decades since the war ended, its reverberations continue to plague the country. Negative trends in the country's economy have thwarted efforts to repair the massive damages that the war visited upon its water and sanitation systems. Landmines that litter the countryside continue to prevent access to natural sources of water for rural dwellers. These problems are compounded by institutional ineptitude. For instance, coordination among actors in the water and sanitation policy field is almost non-existent at both the national and provincial levels (UNICEF, 2008). Uganda has also experienced violent conflicts with far-reaching implications for access to improved water and sanitation in the recent past. In fact, some of the conflicts are ongoing. The most affected areas are the country's southwestern, northern and eastern regions. These regions have known violent conflicts for almost two decades. The consequences of this have been massive internal displacement of populations. Most of the displaced people often sought refuge in excessively crowded refugee camps, where access to improved water and sanitation facilities is extremely limited.

*Droughts and other natural hazards*

The natural environment is at once a blessing and a curse for the Eastern and Southern Africa region (see e.g., UNICEF, 2008). The region's natural threats are a function of several factors. The most prominent of these factors are extremities in climate and rainfall variability. These conditions have been exacerbated in recent times by climate change and related factors. The many consequences of these developments have included growing water scarcity, shrinkage action in natural bodies of water and deforestation. A number of specific examples serve to illustrate this growing problem in the region. Consider the case of Angola. The country enjoys an abundance of rainfall, and boasts vast surface water resources in some parts. At the same time, some portions of the country are semi-arid while others are too rugged and largely inaccessible. Ethiopia, Eritrea, Kenya, and Zambia are some of the countries that have had to wrestle with problems of droughts in the region. In Eritrea, the problem has affected at least two-thirds of the country. Water levels in the affected areas have fallen to an all-time low. Many water sources have actually dried up. These factors jointly account for the fact that the safe water coverage in the country is only about 30 per cent. Kenya typifies the region's extremities. On the one hand, some parts, such as the northern and hinterland areas experience frequent droughts. On the other hand, the Lake and coastal areas are hosts to excessive floods. Both extreme conditions have far-reaching implications for water and sanitation initiatives in the country. In particular, the conditions have tended to strain the country's physically and functionally obsolete water and sanitation infrastructure. Malawi's situation is a little different. The country has not suffered any significant problems of drought in the recent past. In fact, it boasts abundant surface and groundwater resources. However, rapidly growing populations and deforestation are jointly exerting severe pressure on the aquifers of certain parts of the country (UNICEF, 2008). Finally, there is the case of Zambia. Here, the problem is one of declining rainfall. This problem, according to the United Nations Children's Fund, has been steadily worsening during the last

30 years. Resulting from this has been a recurrent drought pattern. This pattern has negatively affected water supply efforts in the country during the last two decades.

*Politics*

It is true that nature has dealt many parts of the Eastern and Southern Africa region a difficult hand. However, it would be erroneous to attribute all of the region's water and sanitation problems to difficult hydrology and vulnerability to natural disasters. To be sure, a significant proportion of the problems is attributable to human actions. Human action, and not nature, is required to harness extant resources to produce, store and distribute water to human settlements. Similarly, human action, and not nature is required to develop sustainable sanitation facilities as well as promote hygienic human behaviour. Failures in this regard are easily traceable to politics, and especially power struggles and the socio-economic inequalities that such struggles engender.

The reverberating effects on water and sanitation of the 2007–2008 Kenyan political crisis continue to be felt in most parts of the country today. The crisis erupted upon the declaration of the incumbent, Mai Kibaki, and not his rival, Raila Odinga, as victor in the presidential election. The violent rampage, which ensued, targeted members of Kibaki's Kikuyu tribe living outside their indigenous homeland. In effect, Kikuyu people, their communities, and especially real estate property throughout the country were the targets of violent attacks. Carcasses of Kikuyu-owned buildings and other structures victimized by the crisis remain unrepaired and now serve as hideouts for criminals in some Kenyan towns. A significant part of the water and sanitation infrastructure in these towns sustained collateral damage as a result of the violence.

Zimbabwe is another country that has suffered political crisis in the region in the recent past. The country is on record for undertaking a number of significant reforms in the water and sanitation sector in the 1990s. One important product of these reforms is the Zimbabwe National Water Authority (ZINWA). This entity was charged with the responsibility of managing the country's water resources. However, its effectiveness has been greatly compromised by political instability and related issues. Particularly, tensions between the country's political rivals have resulted in many posts in the water and sanitation sector remaining vacant. In addition, the economic problems engendered by the country's unstable political situation have resulted in the poor maintenance and disrepair of water and sanitation infrastructure. Furthermore, the highly controversial farm seizure programmes of the country's political leadership led to disruptions in agricultural production and internal displacements. These developments have had significant negative consequences for efforts to improve water and sanitation conditions throughout the country.

## Understanding and dealing with hygiene and sanitation issues

The immediate-post-colonial period in the Southern and Eastern Africa region was marked by mass rural-to-urban migration. For a brief while, the sanitation infrastructure inherited from the colonial era appeared to be adequate. However, with the passage of time, the infrastructure began to show signs of wear and tear. By the 1970s, rapid rates of urban growth, and failure on the part of post-colonial authorities to augment the inventory of sanitation facilities inherited from the colonial era had already conspired to aggravate urban sanitation conditions throughout the region. In efforts to address the problem, local and national governments have collaborated with international entities such as WHO, UNICEF, UN-Habitat, UNDP, and the World Bank to formulate and implement public health improvement programmes. The following paragraphs discuss some of the most prominent of these programmes.

In the 1990s WHO, World Bank and UNDP joined forces to promote "participatory hygiene and sanitation transformation" (PHAST) (World Bank/UNDP, 1998). This strategy deserves more than passing attention here because of its participatory component, which is likely to render it more sustainable than other alternatives. The importance of participation cannot be overstated in matters such as hygiene and sanitation that involve social behaviour and community norms. The World Bank/UNDP and WHO-initiated PHAST was launched initially in 1993 and piloted in six countries in the region. The avowed aim of the pilot phase was to disseminate the methodology and to set the stage for further development (World Bank/UNDP, 1998). PHAST has been defined as a methodology that seeks to promote the participatory learning of practices and techniques that can help communities improve their hygiene behaviours. It is believed that this will result in preventing communicable diseases such as diarrhea, dysentery and cholera. These diseases are typically caused by unhygienic behaviours and surroundings (WSSC, 2009). In other words, the most common life-threatening diseases in the sub-region are related directly or indirectly to sanitation and hygiene. A number of other hygiene related diseases that can be commonly found in the region include skin and eye infections. Preventing or combating these diseases requires not only environmental modifications but also, and perhaps more importantly, changes in individual behaviours. Such changes may include cultivating the habit of regularly washing one's hands, tidying one's surroundings and maintaining general principles of hygiene.

A principal objective of PHAST is to empower communities to carter to their own hygiene and sanitation needs. Therefore, it assumes that, when communities become aware, they are likely to meaningfully contribute to efforts to address their own sanitation needs. PHAST also seeks to enhance the self-esteem of the members of target communities by involving them in the planning process. This aspect of the strategy ensures that members of communities are, and view themselves as, owners of local hygiene and sanitation projects and programmes.

The six countries that were piloted in the programme include Botswana, Ethiopia, Kenya, Uganda, and Zimbabwe.

As articulated in 1998, PHAST was anything but novel. Rather, it was an adaptation of an earlier participatory method known as "Self-esteem Associative Strengths, Resourcefulness Action planning and Responsibility" (SARAR). The avowed aim of this programme, which was adopted by PHAST is to empower community members in a participatory process. In practice, it seeks to, among other things, assess people's knowledge base as well as the potentials and limitations of the local environment. Within the framework of the programme, this is considered an initial step in the process of adopting and implementing an acceptable programme of action.

As this chapter shows, the hygiene and sanitation needs of the Eastern and Southern Africa region are plentiful. Some of the needs, such as those shown on Table 7.1 are quantifiable. Others are not. The quality of data of the quantifiable genre is often questionable. This is especially true for statistics on sanitation coverage in rural areas. The quality of the data notwithstanding, the prevalence of diseases such as diarrhea, dysentery, and cholera that are often associated with insalubrious conditions is indisputable. Success in reversing this situation is contingent upon two factors. The first is the ability to appreciate the multiple dimensions of sanitation problems. The second is the extent to which the source of sanitation and related problems can be accurately identified.

It is erroneous to attribute all hygiene and sanitation problems to a lack of resources. To do so is to be reductionist. The absence of improved sanitation facilities is a function of several factors. Some of these factors may be cultural as opposed to economic in nature. Similarly, failure to adhere to basic norms of hygiene may be unrelated to people's poverty status. Rather, this and other problems may result from simple lack of knowledge. In this case, resolving the problems would entail very little more than educating the people and instituting a series of simple behaviour modifications. To be sure, authorities in the region appear well aware of this. This is evidenced by the results of recent efforts to identify and deal with the sanitation problems that ail the region. For instance, authorities in Botswana, Kenya, Mozambique, Tanzania, Uganda, Zimbabwe are unified in adopting measures to promote the following hygienic behaviours:

- Hand-washing;
- Safe excreta disposal;
- Safe disposal of domestic waste;
- Outdoor and indoor cleanliness; and
- Personal hygiene.

Authorities in Zimbabwe developed an even longer list that includes kitchen hygiene, access to, and use of, protected water supplies.

Except in a few instances such as those involving the construction of improved sanitation and/or water supply facilities, none of the foregoing measures require any significant financial input. Rather, these hygienic practices require simply reminding the population, through public education, of the need to observe common-sense rules of proper sanitation and hygiene. The following mural on a school wall in the region says it all when it comes to the importance of hand-washing as an element of hygiene: "Your health is the Cleanliness of your hands." Failure to make the necessary behaviour modifications has produced catastrophic health consequences in the past (UNDP/World Bank, 1998). For instance, a cholera outbreak wreaked havoc on Tanzania in 1997. Uganda, where poor water and sanitation account for 50 per cent of infant mortality, was dealt a similar blow in the same year. Cholera outbreaks were also reported in Kenya, Zimbabwe, and Mozambique in that same year. In Mozambique, cholera outbreaks are known to mimic the rainfall cycle. Thus, it is safe to infer that the problem is a function of poor drainage facilities. Mozambique is also particularly worthy of special note because it sits at the bottom of the region's improved sanitation ladder. In fact, only 21 per cent of the country's population has access to such facilities (UNDP/World Bank, 1998).

## Conclusion

This chapter has attempted to paint a vivid picture of the hygiene and sanitation problematic in the Eastern and Southern Africa Region. This region is comprised of disparate countries that differ in terms of geographic and demographic size. Yet, they share one thing in common—they are erstwhile European colonies. Two notable exceptions are Ethiopia and Eritrea, which were never officially colonized. However, their sanitation, hygiene and cognate policies were just as externally driven as those of their peers, which are typically classified as erstwhile colonies. Thus, it is safe to say that the sanitation, hygiene and cognate policies of countries in the region, whether officially colonized or not have a common denominator. They were, and continue to be, influenced by European powers. The similarities amongst the countries go beyond their colonial legacy or externally driven policies. They tend to experience the same types of hygiene and sanitation problems. Some of these problems can be dealt with by simple behaviour-changing initiatives such as hand-washing, the safe disposal of human and domestic wastes, outdoor and indoor cleanliness, and so on. Others, such as the safe disposal of chemical and industrial wastes, and the construction of sanitation infrastructure such as sewerage systems, require financial and other resources. These problems are not evenly distributed in space in African urban centres. Arguably the most promising strategy to promote hygiene and sanitation involves establishing and enforcing relevant urban planning rules and regulations. In most cases, these rules and regulations already exist. However, they are not sustainable because they were crafted with different contexts in mind and simply transplanted to Africa. Also worth noting is the uneven distribution of sanitation problems in the region. The disparities exist both at the international and national level. The latter implies differences among districts within the same country. While some districts have more than their own share of hygiene and sanitation problems, others enjoy standards that favourably compare with those in the developed world. The problem of inequitable distribution of sanitation and other infrastructure and service is a function of the colonialism. Colonial hygiene and sanitation schemes sought to address the health needs of European enclaves to the exclusion of native settlements. Thus, any meaningful efforts to address the problem must first and foremost seek to redress these disparities.

# Chapter 8

# Hygiene and Sanitation in Northern Africa

## Introduction

Most international geo-political classification schemes situate North Africa in the Middle-East or Arab World. The geo-administrative classification schemata developed by the World Health Organization (WHO) and the United Nations Children's Fund (UNICEF) deviates from this convention. Within the framework of the WHO/UNICEF schema, Northern Africa, in its entirety, is located within the continent of Africa. The region comprises five sovereign countries, namely Egypt, Sudan, Morocco, Algeria, Tunisia, Libya and Western Sahara. Sixty-two million people live in this region, which is the most urbanized in Africa (WHO/UNICEF, 2008).

This chapter focuses on the hygiene and sanitation situation in the region. The chapter takes off in the next section by presenting pertinent background information on the region. A significant portion of the section is dedicated to examining the influences of Western urban planning principles and philosophy on spatial organization in this region. The aim is to promote understanding of the impact of such influences on the region's hygiene and sanitation conditions. A subsequent section provides an overview of these conditions in contemporary perspective. Some time is spent assessing the region's progress towards hygiene and sanitation-related targets of the Millennium Development Goals (MDGs). Next, the focus is turned to specific major cities within the region. This is intended to provide a close-up picture of the region's urban hygiene and sanitation problematic.

## Northern Africa region: background

As stated above, the Northern Africa region as delineated by WHO/UNICEF consists of five sovereign nations (see Figure 8.1). These include Egypt, Sudan, Morocco, Algeria, Tunisia, Libya and Western Sahara. Western Sahara, for which statistics are unavailable, is excluded from further discussion here. A common thread running through the development profile of these countries is the fact that they are significantly wealthier than their sub-Saharan neighbours. This provides at least partial explanation for their emergence as the only African countries on track to meet the hygiene-and-sanitation-related targets of the MDGs. This subject is revisited before concluding the chapter. For now, it is important to pay attention to another common feature of the countries comprising Northern Africa.

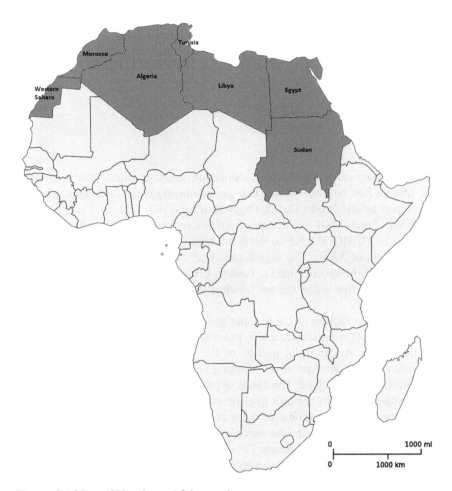

**Figure 8.1 Map of Northern Africa region**

*Source*: Author's rendition based on blank map from the 'freely-licensed educational media content' world wide website, Wikimedia Commons at http://commons.wikimedia.rg/wiki/category:blank_maps_of_Africa.

Like their sub-Saharan neighbours, Northern African countries were subjected to European colonialism. However, unlike their sub-Saharan African neighbours, Northern African countries were psychologically conditioned to resent Western intrusion and acculturation (Bartleby.com, Online). Thus, one would have expected to find hardly any traces of European influence in the region. However, this is not the case. In fact, visible marks of European influences can be seen on the built environment throughout the region. It is necessary to note that the region is replete with ancient cities. These cities had developed sophisticated spatial structures complete with complex pieces of hygiene and sanitation infrastructure. These pieces of infrastructure were supplanted by facilities of European origin beginning in the early-19th century. This period coincides with the onset of the European colonial era in the region. By the late-19th century, most of Northern Africa had been colonized by one or another European power. In this regard, Algeria, Tunisia and Morocco became colonies or protectorates of France in 1830, 1881 and 1912 respectively. Britain took control of Egypt as a colony in 1882, and Sudan in 1899. Italian colonial reign in Libya began in 1911.

Efforts to introduce Western principles of hygiene and sanitation in Northern Africa are particularly noteworthy for two reasons. First, they were ideologically driven. Second, they were intended to achieve political objectives. This latter point deserves further elaboration. It is no secret that European powers viewed colonization as a vehicle for getting back at the Ottoman Empire, which had humiliated them earlier on (cf., Ayataç, 2007). Accordingly, European powers proceeded with unmatched gusto to modernize the built environment and commensurate institutions in the region. In this regard, European colonial authorities moved speedily to overlay customary systems of land tenure, municipal governance, including hygiene and sanitation, with Euro-centric varieties.

To reiterate a point made earlier, Northern Africa had a very strong urban tradition that pre-dated the European colonial era by centuries. This, especially the presence of well developed and densely populated cities, complete with circumscribing walls, posed significant problems to European city builders. Consequently, rather than alter existing urban structures, colonial planners in the region set out to develop new towns or cities based on European principles of urban design (Christopher, 1984). These new towns or what the French called, *villes nouvelles*, were created to serve as exclusive European enclaves. Thus, as was commonplace throughout sub-Saharan Africa, racial residential segregation was also the norm in Northern Africa. However, it is necessary to underscore the fact that what obtained in North Africa was de facto racial residential segregation. This is because segregation was never officially a planning policy in colonial North Africa. One exception, that having to do with the *medinas* in Morocco, is noteworthy here. A 1917 decree by Marshal Hubert Lyautey (1854–1934), while he was the Resident-General in Morocco, forbade Europeans to live in the *medinas* (Christopher, 1984: 177).

In Algeria, Tunisia and Morocco, these new towns reflected French urban planning style. The towns were designed to promote French notions of aesthetics and respond to hygiene, sanitation as well as public health needs. With respect to the former objective, the towns were furnished with broad straight boulevards separating city blocks, minor feeder streets and plots dividing the blocks and high density multi-storey buildings enclosed within central terraces. The inclusion of these features was part of an effort to replicate Georges Eugene Haussmann's design of Paris in colonial North Africa (UN, 2009). Efforts to attain the latter objective included, but were not limited to, requiring strict adherence to Western-style building codes, and the containment of animals within well secured fences.

In addition to the introduction of Western spatial design principles, colonial authorities also crafted growth management policies to control the expansion of human settlements. One effect of this was to constrain the physical expansion of the older settlements, that is, the areas that were occupied by members of the indigenous populations. Thus, the demographic growth of these areas, particularly the *medinas*, was never matched by commensurate spatial expansion. Policies of this genre can be logically viewed as constituting the main source of many health problems in the built environment in the region. This assertion is bolstered by empirical evidence. For instance, by the 1930s natural growth had occasioned overcrowding in many of the *medinas* in the region (Christopher, 1984; UN, 2009). Rural immigrants in search of greener pastures in the growing and increasingly economically vibrant cities were compelled to seek accommodation in already overcrowded walled indigenous settlements.

However, with the passage of time, and in violation of planning legislation in vogue at the time, they began squatting on the fringes of built-up areas. These new settlements, which were typically composed of housing units of the makeshift variety, marked the onset of informal settlement or *biddonvilles* in the region. Considering such settlements a threat to public health, colonial authorities initially embarked on demolishing them. Later on, they realized that efforts to eradicate the settlements constituted an exercise in futility. Accordingly, they moved instead to improve the increasingly unbearable conditions in the settlements. The informal settlements were marked by the absence of basic hygiene and sanitation services. Colonial authorities thus sought to reverse the situation by introducing basic Western-style hygiene and sanitation facilities. This essentially marked a policy change. Prior to World War II, colonial authorities in the region were concerned exclusively with the hygiene and sanitation needs of European enclaves. Improved medical knowledge suggested that contagious water and airborne diseases could be communicated from the *medinas* and informal settlements to European enclaves. This occasioned a broadening of colonial government hygiene and sanitation policies to encompass all human settlements in the region.

## Sanitation coverage in Northern Africa

Northern Africa is the only region on the continent to be rated as 'on track' to meet the hygiene and sanitation targets of the Millennium Development Goals (MDGs). In fact, the region is said to be the only in the entire developing world that has already surpassed the sanitation-related MDG targets (WHO/UNICEF, 2009). This means one or both of the following. First, for any given country in the region, hygiene and sanitation coverage is less than 5 per cent below the rate that country needed to reach the MDG target. Second, sanitation coverage is 95 per cent or higher. As Table 8.1 shows, only a small proportion of Northern Africans use unimproved sanitation facilities (WHO/UNICEF, 2008). Another way of appreciating the region's distinguished record on hygiene and sanitation is to chart trends in this regard during the last couple of decades. As Table 8.1 shows, the region has registered significant gains in sanitation conditions during

**Table 8.1 Progress in sanitation coverage in Northern Africa, 1990–2006**

| Year | Sanitation coverage | | | | | | | |
|---|---|---|---|---|---|---|---|---|
| | Urban (%) | | | | Rural (%) | | | |
| | Improved | Shared | Unimproved | Open Defecation | Improved | Shared | Unimproved | Open Defecation |
| 1990 | 79 | 6 | 13 | 3 | 40 | 5 | 21 | 35 |
| 2000 | 82 | 6 | 9 | 3 | 47 | 7 | 22 | 25 |
| 2006 | 84 | 6 | 8 | 3 | 51 | 7 | 23 | 19 |

*Source:* Compiled from WHO/UNICEF (2008).

this period. In 1990 the proportion of urban residents with access to improved sanitation in the region stood at 79 per cent. A decade later in 2000, this proportion rose, albeit slightly, to 82 per cent. By 2006 the proportion had increased to 84 per cent. However, the proportion of the urban population using shared sanitation facilities remained constant at six per cent from 1990 to 2006. Numerically, as many as 89 to 99 million urban inhabitants in the region have access to improved sanitation facilities. Proportionately, however, the relevant values have remained constant. These statistics tend to belie reality. To appreciate this line of reasoning, it is necessary to understand that the urban population of the region has been growing steadily. Thus, while the proportion of the population depending on shared sanitation facilities has remained constant, the absolute number has significantly increased.

A stark contrast exists between urban and rural areas in the region when it comes to sanitation coverage. As the Joint Monitoring Programme (JMP) noted, urban residents in the region are one-and-a-half times more likely to have sanitation than rural residents (JMP, 2008). Thus, as is the case throughout the rest of Africa, sanitation coverage is significantly lower in rural than in urban areas. In rural areas, the proportion of residents with access to improved sanitation was 40 per cent in 1990. In 2000 this proportion had grown to 47 per cent. In 2006 the proportion stood at 51 per cent.

Another set of statistics worthy of note is related to the proportion of the population in urban and rural areas that use unimproved sanitation facilities. The proportion of the urban population depending on unimproved sanitation has significantly decreased since 1990. In 1990 this proportion was 13 per cent. It dropped to 9 per cent in 2000. Half a decade later in 2006 there was yet another slight decrease to 8 per cent. In rural areas, the picture of unimproved sanitation facility usage is paradoxical. While the statistics improved significantly on all fronts, rural dependence on unimproved sanitation facilities grew worse between 1990 and 2006. In this regard, the proportion of the rural population depending on unimproved sanitation facilities rose, albeit marginally, from 21 to 22 per cent between 1990 and 2000. This proportion grew from 22 to 23 per cent between 2000 and 2006.

**Table 8.2 Sanitation conditions in the Northern Africa region**

| Country | Population (x 1,000) | Urban (%) | | | | Rural (%) | | | |
|---|---|---|---|---|---|---|---|---|---|
| | | Improved | Shared | Unimproved | Open defecation | Improved | Shared | Unimproved | Open defecation |
| Algeria | 34373 | 98 | n/a | 1 | 1 | 88 | n/a | 2 | 10 |
| Egypt | 81527 | 97 | 3 | 0 | 0 | 92 | 6 | 2 | 0 |
| Libya | n/a | n/a | n/a | n/a | n/a | n/a | n/a | n/a | n/a |
| Morocco | 31606 | 83 | 14 | 3 | 0 | 52 | 6 | 4 | 38 |
| Sudan | 41348 | 55 | n/a | 25 | 20 | 18 | n/a | 24 | 58 |
| Tunisia | 10169 | 96 | 2 | 2 | 0 | 64 | 8 | 14 | 14 |
| Western Sahara | n/a | n/a | n/a | n/a | n/a | n/a | n/a | n/a | n/a |

*Source:* Based on data from WHO/UNICEF (2010).

Even more ironic are the statistics relating to open defecation. About as much as three per cent of the urban population in Northern Africa practices open defecation. This percentage remained constant from 1990 to 2006. Numerically, however, the number of people practicing open defecation in the region dropped significantly from 27 million in 1990 to 18 million in 2006.

A clearer picture of sanitation conditions in Northern Africa emerges with a disaggregation of the relevant data. On Table 8.2, the disaggregation has been done on a country-by-country basis. As the table shows, Algeria's 98 per cent access to improved sanitation facilities for urban residents is the highest in the region. Sudan, where only 55 per cent of urban residents have access to improved sanitation facilities, trails all countries in the region on this score. The country is also unique with as much as 20 per cent of urban residents practicing open defecation in a region where such a practice is extremely rare. However, open defecation is not as rare in rural areas. Up to 20 per cent of rural residents in Algeria practice open defecation. This is noteworthy given that almost all urban-based Algerians have access to improved sanitation facilities. If nothing else, this accentuates the problem of urban bias in infrastructure provisioning that is a defining characteristic of developing nations. Yet, Algeria ranks best with respect to open defecation for rural residents in comparison to other countries in the region. Again, Sudan, with a majority (58%) of rural residents practicing open defecation, lays claim to the worst record.

## Access to water

North Africa is significantly more urbanized than Africa south of the Sahara. As Table 8.3 shows, with the exception of Egypt and Sudan, the majority of people in the region live in urban centres. Even then, urbanization levels in Egypt (43%) and Sudan (40%) are higher than that of most countries in sub-Sahara Africa. With as much as 78 per cent of its population based in urban areas, Libya is the most urbanized country in Northern Africa. Countries in the region are relatively better off than their sub-Saharan African neighbours with respect to access to improved water. Water service coverage in almost all urban centres in the region is a hundred per cent or close. For instance, as Table 8.3 shows, all residents of Cairo, the largest city in the region, have access to water services. With only 54 per cent of its urban residents boasting access to improved water facilities, Libya trails all countries in the region on this score. Yet, it must be noted that Libya is unique in this regard. The proportion (55%) of rural residents is greater than the proportion (54%) of urbanites with access to improved water sources. At the same time, it has the highest proportion (46%) of total rural residents who must make do with unimproved water facilities. Again, Egypt leads all of its regional peers in terms of access to improved water sources for rural residents. Only four per cent of the country's rural residents is compelled to fetch water from what may be classified as an unimproved source.

**Table 8.3 Access to improved sources of water in Northern Africa, 2008**

| Country | Surface area (km²) | Percent urban pop. | Improved Water (%) | | | Unimproved Water (%) | | |
|---|---|---|---|---|---|---|---|---|
| | | | Urban | Rural | Total | Urban | Rural | Total |
| Algeria | 2,381,741 | 66 | 85 | 79 | 83 | 15 | 21 | 17 |
| Egypt | 2,665 | 43 | 100 | 98 | 99 | 0 | 4 | 1 |
| Libya | 1,759,540 | 78 | 54 | 55 | 54 | 46 | 45 | 46 |
| Morocco | 446,550 | 58 | 98 | 60 | 81 | 2 | 40 | 19 |
| Sudan | 1,861,484 | 40 | 64 | 52 | 57 | 36 | 48 | 43 |
| Tunisia | 163,610 | 67 | 99 | 84 | 94 | 1 | 16 | 6 |
| W. Sahara | 266,000 | 82 | n/a | n/a | n/a | n/a | n/a | n/a |

*Source:* UNICEF (2010) and CIA (online).

## Institutional context

The institutional context for water and sanitation policy making in Northern Africa is dominated by state or public agencies. Private entities tend to play a relatively less significant role. However, Morocco is exceptional in this regard. Here, as Box 8.1 shows, private for-profit corporations are very active in the water and sanitation sector. As we have already noted, the Northern Africa region has made significant progress in the water and sanitation domain. Despite this achievement, the region faces a number of daunting challenges. These challenges are in large part of an institutional nature. The most prominent of these challenges were chronicled by the Global Water Partnership's (GWP) initiative in the Mediterranean Region in 2008. The most prominent of these challenges have been identified and discussed by the Organization for Economic Co-operation and Development (OECD), and are summarized below (see GWP, 2008; OECD, 2010).

### Box 8.1 Private participation in the water sector in Morocco

In a way, the participation of private entities in the water domain in Morocco is a colonial legacy. During the colonial era, private concessions ran the entire territory. However, soon after the demise of the colonial era, indigenous authorities decided to nationalize all private utility corporations. In the mid-1990s these corporations were once more privatized. Two particular private French-based corporations were the earliest and best known to secure water concessions in the country. The first is *Lyonnaise des Eaux*, which later became known as SUEZ. It was awarded the Casablanca concession in 1997, and that of Rabat the following year. The second is *Veolia Environnement*. It was awarded concessions in Tangiers and Tetouan. By 2009, private utility corporations provided water and sanitation services to 38 per cent of the country's urban residents. Privatization of the water and sanitation sector in Morocco has been without opposition. Several aspects of the privatization plan, (e.g., sale of public utility companies and lowering of trade tariffs), have been controversial. Government authorities contend that the country's water resources are increasingly depleting, and only the 'free market' is capable of managing scarcity. Opponents counter, arguing that privatizing water is a prescription for depriving the poor of access to an indispensable public good.

*Source*: Lahlou, M. (Online). "Water Privatization in Morocco: First Lessons Drawn from the Case of Lyonnaise des Eaux in Casablanca." Transnational Institute (TNI). http://www.tni.org/archives/act/18357.

One of the most conspicuous of the institutional problems has to do with the journey from policy formulation to implementation. In this regard, otherwise sound policies for sustainable water management have been enacted throughout most of the region. However, the implementation of these policies has proven to be excruciatingly difficult. One reason for this is that there are no valid monitoring tools. Another, and perhaps the most important reason for this, is the lack of the necessary political will. Policy makers in the region face the unique challenge of striking a delicate balance between religion and realism. For instance, religious dogma views water as a gift from Allah (or God) that cannot be sold or exchanged. However, realism dictates the need for some form of payment for water for the sake of cost recovery if for no other reason.

In addition, there is the absence of strong and enforceable legislation and regulations. Such legislation and regulations are required to address the region's current and future water and sanitation needs. Their absence has meant, among other things that these needs are only insufficiently dealt with. This problem is compounded by yet another problem, that of inadequate financial commitment as well as technical support for the water and sanitation sector.

**Table 8.4 Government ministries in water and sanitation, Northern Africa**

| Country | Ministries with Responsibility in the Water and Sanitation Sector |
|---------|------------------------------------------------------------------|
| Algeria | Ministry of Health, Population & Hospital Reform; Ministry of Housing and Urban Development; Ministry of Water Resources. |
| Egypt | Ministry of Health & Population; Ministry of Housing, Utilities & Urban Communities; Ministry of Irrigation & Water Resources. |
| Libya | Transitional Government (No permanent government in place yet). |
| Morocco | Ministry of Energy, Mines, Water & Environment; Ministry Delegate to the P.M. in charge of Urbanization & Housing; Secretary of State to the Ministry of Energy, Mines, Water & Environment. |
| Sudan | Ministry of Health; Ministry of Irrigation & Water Resources; Ministry of Environment, Forestry & Urban Development. |
| Tunisia | Ministry of Public Health; Ministry of Agriculture and Environment; Ministry of Public Works. |
| W. Sahara | N/A. |

*Source*: Based on data from National Government Websites & CIA World Factbook (www.cia.gov).

Furthermore, countries in the region are uniformly guilty of overloading their public sector. In practice, this means not only an overstaffed bureaucracy but also one that is bloated with too many institutional bodies. Table 8.4 shows what for all practical purposes, is only a tip of the iceberg. As the table shows, there are at least three ministries responsible for overseeing the implementation of water and sanitation policies. However, the problem is not necessarily with the sheer number of ministries operating in the water and sanitation domain. Rather, it has to do with the fact that these entities and their sub-national units have overlapping, and unavoidably confusing responsibilities in the domain. This invariably leads to the unnecessary fragmentation of roles, which in turn leads to resource waste.

**Box 8.2 Multiplicity of entities in Tunisia's water and sanitation sector**

Two major ministerial bodies were in charge of water and sanitation in Tunisia until the revolution that ousted the Zine El Abidine Ben Ali regime on 15 January 2011. Although some ministries were absorbed by others, the water and sanitation domain remains virtually unchanged. Three major ministerial bodies, the Ministry of Agriculture and Environment, the Ministry of Public Works, and the Ministry of Health have major responsibilities in the water and sanitation domain. The Ministry of Agriculture and Environment is responsible for issues relating to the overall supply and use of water. It is also charged with the responsibility for impact studies and monitoring of environment systems. Other institutional actors in the water sector include the Commission of Public Hydraulic Domain and the National Water Council. These two latter are charged with the responsibility of assisting the ministerial bodies in the water and sanitation domain. In addition, two centralized, public autonomous agencies are in charge of managing the country's water and sanitation systems. One of these agencies is the National Water Development and Distribution Company known under its French acronym, SONEDE (i.e., *Société Nationale d'Exploitation et de Distribution des Eaux*). For a long time subsequent to its creation in 1968, this agency has been responsible for building, operating and maintaining the country's water infrastructure exclusively in urban areas. However, it had recently extended its operations into rural areas. There is yet another autonomous public agency in the country's water and sanitation domain. It is the National Sanitation Bureau, known under its French acronym, ONAS (i.e., *Office Nationale d'Assainissement)*. It has been responsible for sewage collection, treatment and disposal in the country since 1974. Since 2004 it has operated under the supervisory authority of the Ministry of Environment and Sustainable Development. Furthermore, there have always been two additional public agencies in the country's water and sanitation domain. The one is the General Directorate for Major Waterworks (i.e., *Direction générale des grands travaux hydrauliques*). The other is the Directorate for Rural Engineering and Water Resource Development (i.e., *Direction générale du genie rural et de l'exploitation des eaux*). The former is in charge of constructing large dams and irrigation infrastructure. The latter is responsible for water resource management, irrigation and sanitation in rural areas.

*Source*: OECD (2010).

Then, there is the problem of cost. The cost of creating and maintaining a sound water governance system can be prohibitively high even for an oil-rich nation such as Libya. This cost has been estimated to be in the millions of Euros (OECD, 2010: 297). The cost is associated with the following: 1) developing national and local plans; 2) establishing and operating coordinating mechanisms and new national and local institutions; 3) training and capacity building; and 4) stakeholder consultation. The multiplicity of institutional actors also tends to aggravate problems such as corruption, which constitutes a defining characteristic of developing countries.

Yet another institutional problem confronting the water and sanitation sector in the region is the dire shortage of skilled labour power. This has often dictated a need to import foreign labour input in efforts to execute water projects in the region. For example, Libya's Great Man-Made River (GMMR) Project depended on skilled labour power from South Korea, Japan, the US, the UK and Germany for its execution. On its face the importation of skilled labour may appear beneficial to the recipient nation. However, upon closer examination, this often turns out not to be the case. Such importation creates unnecessary dependency by the recipient country on the exporting country. In this regard, skilled labour power must be imported to carry out the basic repairs and maintenance chores necessary for water or sanitation system functioning.

A related problem is the lack of complete, valid and reliable data that can serve as input in water and sanitation decision making processes. The problem is exacerbated by the fact that extant data collection and monitoring programmes involve too many entities. The multiplicity of these entities is in and of itself not a problem. The nagging problem concerns the fact that they operate without any sort of coordination and/or integration mechanism. The absence of coordination amongst entities within a common policy field is a prescription of chaos. Entities operating under such conditions are inescapably dysfunctional as they tend to work at cross-purposes with each other.

Another endemic institutional problem in the region is the tendency to exclude primary beneficiaries of public infrastructure projects from the decision making process. With the citizen uprisings, christened the 'Arab Spring,' that have recently taken place in the region, some change may be in the making. However, until such change becomes reality, we know that the participation of local stakeholders has never been accorded any importance in the region. Yet, unless the input of all stakeholders is enlisted, the success of water, sanitation and cognate projects is seldom guaranteed. Participation by local actors and stakeholders is critical for project sustainability. When these actors and stakeholders are involved in the decision making process, they are likely to support the project and ensure its sustenance once it has been implemented. Yet, the potential contribution of project primary beneficiaries goes beyond ensuring the project's sustenance. They can be counted upon to provide invaluable locally-derived and experience-based knowledge necessary for the project's success from conception through formulation to implementation.

**Natural and man-made constraints**

Factors mitigating against efforts to improve access to improved water and sanitation facilities in Northern Africa are mainly of the natural variety. The geographically larger countries in the region stretch from the Mediterranean Sea in the north to the Sahara Desert in the south. Thus, most of the region is desert with a litany of geological conditions that have far-reaching implications for water supply. These conditions are aggravated by man-made calamities, particularly war. In addition, there are problems that are rooted in a variety of institutional factors.

*Geological and other natural difficulties*

Northern African countries face daunting problems resulting from their difficult natural environment. Soil erosion, often caused by overgrazing and poor farming practices, is commonplace. In some countries such as Algeria, this problem is aggravated by desertification. The country's dams are frequently clogged by silt and mud. On its part, Egypt's geological make-up exposes the country to natural disasters such as droughts, earthquakes, flash floods, landslide, and sandstorms. In some of the countries, the desert poses several problems. This is the case with Libya, which is 90 per cent desert. In such situations freshwater resources are extremely limited to non-existent. Libya is fortunate to have been blessed with an ample supply of oil. Huge sums of money from oil sales have enabled the country to invest in the Great Man-Made River Project. This is the most extensive such scheme in the world. It provides some 6.5 million cubic meters of water a day free of charge to residents of major Libyan cities such as Benghazi, Sirte and Tripoli as well as smaller towns throughout the country. Sudan faces persistent droughts that tend to constrain the provisioning of potable water and sanitation facilities. Morocco's mountainous northern region is geologically unstable and prone to earthquakes and periodic droughts that also thwart similar efforts in that country.

*Man-made disasters*

Many of the problems thwarting efforts to address the water and sanitation needs in Northern Africa are of the man-made variety. These include the improper disposal of raw sewage, petroleum refining wastes and industrial effluents, poor agricultural practices and war. The improper disposal of waste or dumping is a leading cause of water pollution in the region. In this regard, the Mediterranean Sea is increasingly polluted by petroleum wastes, soil erosion and fertilizer runoff. In addition, there are underground water pollution problems engendered by agricultural pesticides, raw sewage and industrial effluents. These problems are aggravated by inadequate management of scarce water resources.

A leading man-made factor with far-reaching implications for water and sanitation is war. A good manifestation of the impact of war on water and sanitation facilities is presented by the recently concluded armed conflict in

Libya. The less than one-year brief conflict was between forces loyal to the late Colonel Muammar Gaddafi and those of the Transitional Government backed by NATO. Although brief, the conflict severely damaged the country's fragile water and sanitation infrastructure. Gaddafi loyalist are said to have destroyed water pumps and attacked engineers attempting to restart pumping stations of the Great Man-Made River (GMMR) Project. This resulted in the disconnection of water supply to Tripoli and other human settlements in the capital city region. NATO air forces were accused of bombing a pipe supply factory in Brega. This factory was responsible for servicing the GMMR project. If such interruptions to water services did not result in many tragic outcomes, it is because of the role UNICEF and the World Food Programme (WFP) played. These two international development agencies were active in distributing bottled water through hundreds of local mosques especially in Tripoli, Misrata, Bani Walid and Sirte. Armed conflicts ended with the capture and dead of Gaddafi on 20 October 2011, and the war was declared officially over three days later. However, it will take some time for the country's severely damaged water and sanitation infrastructure to be repaired.

## Hygiene and sanitation in Cairo, Egypt

With a population of 18 million, Cairo emerges, by far, as the most populous city in Northern Africa. Unlike most cities in Africa, Cairo has a history that dates back to antiquity. It is the capital city of Egypt, which arguably lays claim to one of the richest histories in the world. Archaeological data suggest that ancient Egypt boasted well-designed sophisticated and complex sanitation systems. Ancient Egyptian human settlements came complete with meticulously designed drainage systems, public toilets, and even public bath houses. Yet, municipal authorities in these ancient settlements wrestled with hygiene and sanitation problems that were less challenging than those faced by their contemporary counterparts.

Current hygiene and sanitation conditions in Cairo can be better appreciated within the broader context of Egypt as a whole. In line with other Northern African countries, Egypt has registered enormous achievements in water coverage (WHO/UNICEF, 2008). In 1990 as much as 89 per cent of urban households had access to piped water. By 2006, the country had attained almost universal coverage (99%) with respect to pipe borne water in urban areas. Coverage with respect to water supply rose from 39 to 82 per cent in rural areas between 1990 and 2006. Another achievement relates to open defecation, which has been completely eliminated in urban areas.

Yet, the country faces challenges in a number of areas. Prominent in this regard, are the deficiencies that characterize the country's sanitation sector. The country has a very limited central sewerage system, which is confined to the urban areas. In fact, this system serves no more than a third of the population (Sharabas, 2010). Also, sanitation facilities, including those for treating wastewater, are antiquated and malfunctioning. In fact, more than 95 per cent of rural areas throughout the country have no wastewater treatment and collection facilities at all (Abdel-Halim et al., 2008: 1456). Domestic wastewater in rural Egypt is treated mainly in septic tanks. This is not to say that conventional wastewater treatment plants are completely absent in the country. To be sure, there are more than 200 such plants scattered throughout the country, but mainly concentrated in the urban areas (Ibid). The largest of these plants is located in Gabal el Asfar, to the Northeast of Cairo. Together, the country's wastewater plants treated about 11 million cubic metres per day in 2004 (Sharabas, 2010). The Gabal el Asfar plant alone served more than 6 million people when its first stage was completed in 2004. The millions of cubic metres of treated water this plant discharges are emptied into the Belbeis Drain and then into Bahr El Baqar Drain. This is in turn drained into Lake Manzala, some 170 kilometres from Cairo. However, the severe shortage of functional wastewater treatment plants has resulted in a lot of untreated wastewater being released into the country's main fresh water source, the River Nile. By one estimate, as much as 3.8 billion cubic meters of water is released into the Nile annually. Out of this, only 35 per cent is considered properly treated.

Sanitation coverage remains low, especially in the rural areas. Consequently, in such areas, dependence on unimproved sanitation facilities, including holes in the ground, bushes, and other unacceptable systems remains significantly high. Municipal sanitation facilities, including centralized sewerage systems are restricted to urban centres, especially the country's two largest cities, Cairo and Alexandria. A report by the Central Department of Lower Egypt Projects, National Organization for Potable Water and Sanitary Drainage, Cairo, contains some very telling data on sanitation in these cities and Egypt in general (see Sharabas, 2010). Cairo, the country's capital and largest city, has the highest sanitation coverage. As much as 77 per cent of the city's population is connected. Sanitation in Alexandria, the second largest city, is lower at 65 per cent. The coverage is significantly lower in the rest of the country. In this regard, about 30 per cent of the people in rural areas receive adequate sanitation services in quantitative and qualitative terms. Also, only 30 per cent of the country's entire population has access to adequate wastewater services. The absence of sanitation and wastewater treatment facilities has had undesirable consequences such as "widespread surface ponding of wastewater and the contamination of drainage channels" (Ibid: 158). These consequences are especially grave for places such as the Delta region, which is characterized by high population density, impervious soils and high groundwater tables. The application of low-cost, onsite sanitation facilities is rendered difficult in such areas.

*Cairo*

It is necessary to examine some of the specific hygiene and sanitation matters relating to Cairo before closing this segment of the present chapter. As stated earlier, almost all (98%) of Cairo's residents have access to pipe borne water.

However, a significantly smaller proportion of the residents of this mega city have access to adequate sanitation facilities. In fact, the city is generally saddled with problems relating to the safe disposal of sewage. Cairo, like other major cities in Northern Africa in particular and Africa in general, is wrestling with common sanitation problems such as garbage collection and disposal. It is true that the Egyptian government and municipal authorities have invested a lot of time and other resources into efforts to eradicate Cairo's hygiene and sanitation problems. Yet, evidence emerging from the city indicates that the efforts have left much to be desired. As recently as 2009, a New York Times article characterized Cairo as a "litter-strewn metropolis" (NYT, 2009, para. 1). The article took aim at Cairo's garbage problem, which had become increasingly nagging in recent years as the mega-city has grown rapidly in demographic and geographic terms. The problem caught the attention of the international community after spring 2009. This is when Egypt faced an eminent threat from swine flu and the country's health authorities mandated the killing of all pigs as a health protection measure. Unbeknownst to these authorities, the measure was not only misguided but produced significant negative consequences for hygiene and sanitation initiatives in Cairo. Box 8.3 contains a more detailed description of these consequences.

The 'garbage problem' that has emerged in Cairo as a result of the misguided massive pig-slaughtering policy in spring 2009 illuminates a more profound problem with sanitation policymaking in developing countries. This problem is discussed in greater detail in the next chapter. For now, suffice to state that the policies are usually top-down, often fail to pay any attention to their consequences, and are typically never followed-up. In the case at hand, a more bottom-up or democratized policymaking approach would have revealed that garbage collection in Cairo has always been an informal sector undertaking. People in Cairo are not used to taking their garbage to the street-side curbs to be picked up by garbage trucks as is the practice in Western societies. Rather, they are accustomed to having their garbage collected from their door steps by people they know. Those who have efficiently and effectively executed this task in Cairo for over half a century are the zabaleen (Arabic for garbage collectors). The zabaleen are members of Egypt's minority Coptic Christian population—only 10 per cent of the country's 70 million inhabitants. They live on the cliffs of the city's eastern edge, and raise pigs for food. Trash has always been their business—and a lucrative business at that. The zabaleen are reputed for their ingenuity in recycling and selling items they meticulously select from the tons of garbage they collect every day. They are also known for feeding the organic waste from these tons of trash to their pigs. These pigs, as stated earlier constitute an important food source for the Christians. Thus, very little in the waste collection process is actually 'wasted.' In fact, according to one source, the garbage collection method involving the zabaleen boasts a recycling rate of no less than 85 per cent (IRP, 2006). In comparison, multinational formal garbage collection companies are required by law to recycle only 20 per cent of the trash they collect (Ibid, para. 16).

## Box 8.3 Pigs as 'sanitation workers' in Cairo

As paradoxical as it may sound, pigs have for a long time served as the most efficient 'sanitation workers' in Cairo, Egypt. Pigs do not complain, they never go on strike, and ask neither for sick leave nor any compensation. Their role in the sanitation domain remained as one of Cairo's best-kept secrets until immediately subsequent to spring 2009. In spring 2009, Egyptian authorities had erroneously incriminated pigs as the vector of the lethal swine flu. All pigs in Egypt were condemned to death and ordered to be killed with immediate effect. The massive killing of pigs as a public policy went largely unchallenged for two main reasons. First, most Egyptians are Muslims and do not eat pork. Only the country's very small Christian minority considers pigs a source of food. Second, the characterization of pigs, albeit erroneously, as a vector of swine flu, made them a health threat. In its misguided massive pig-slaughtering policy, the government was oblivious to the pigs' arguably most important role as 'sanitation workers' in large Egyptian cities such as Cairo. In fact, prior to spring 2009 when the policy was effectively implemented, pigs used to consume tons of organic waste throughout Cairo. Subsequent to the policy's implementation, the sight of rotting food piles on streets in middle-class neighbourhoods such as Heliopolis and in poor districts such as Imbaba, became commonplace. One local resident painted the following picture of the hygiene and sanitation consequences of the policy. Once the pigs were gone, the pathways became terribly littered, garbage heaps could be found everywhere and pungent odour rapidly took over the air. Thus, "what started out as an impulsive response to the swine flu threat has turned into a social, environmental and political problem for the Arab world's most populous nation" (para. 8).

*Source*: New York Times (2009).

However, in its bid to modernize, or more accurately, Westernize, and make Cairo a world-class mega-city, Egyptian authorities have been busy during the last few years with efforts to completely replace the *zabaleen* with formal garbage collection companies. Resulting from these efforts has, among other things, been the hiring of multi-national garbage collection companies. In 2006, it was reported that these companies collected only about one-third of the 13,000 or so tons of trash that Cairo's 18 million residents generate daily (IRP, 2006, para. 10).

### Hygiene and sanitation in Casablanca, Morocco

Casablanca is Morocco's most populous city. Some sources hold that the city is just a little more than 3 million (3,245,000) (e.g., CIA, Online). The wider Casablanca metropolitan area has a population of 4.5 million (a clearer and more meaningful picture of the city's hygiene and sanitation situation can be obtained by discussing the situation within the broader context of Morocco's political economy). Like its regional peers, Morocco has registered many socio-economic gains over the years. It is considered a middle-income country. More noteworthy for the purpose of the present discussion is the fact that Morocco is on track to exceed the water-and-sanitation-related targets of the Millennium Development Goals (MDGs). Access to improved water and sanitation is nearly universal. This achievement is largely a function of sound policy and greater government investments in water and sanitation projects. The government's laudable accomplishments should, however, not veil the fact that significant deficiencies remain especially in the sanitation domain. However, it must be noted that most of the deficiencies are in the rural areas, where 13 out the country's 30 million inhabitants live. Only 56 per cent of the population in these areas has access to piped water. The proportion without access to improved sanitation facilities is significantly less at 35 per cent (World Bank, 2006). Yet, deficiencies in sanitation and related infrastructure and services are not exclusively rural problems in Morocco. Such problems, albeit on a relatively smaller scale, are also present in the country's urban areas, especially the informal and peri-urban settlements. By some accounts, as many as 2 million Moroccans living in such settlements have no access to improved sanitation facilities (Beauchene, 2009).

In Casablanca alone, some 45,000 households comprising 90,000 inhabitants do not receive adequate water supply and sanitation services (Ibid, para. 3). Those particularly without access to these basic services reside in the city's more than 400 shantytowns. Most of these towns are a by-product of the unprecedented population growth and rapid pace of urbanization that Casablanca experienced during the past century. Here, it must be noted that the city jumped from a modest 20,000 inhabitants at the beginning of the century to its current size of 4.5 million (Lydec, online). Today, more than 400,000 people live in such towns, which are mainly located at the fringes of Casablanca. Access to piped water in these towns is ensured only through a few public standpipes. Hence some shantytown residents depend on precarious sources of water such as contaminated shallow wells and prohibitively expensive water vendors. As for sanitation, residents of these towns are compelled to use cesspits or poorly designed septic tanks. These and other forms of unimproved sanitation systems pose serious threats to public health. If nothing else, such systems have a propensity to, among other things, contaminate shallow ground water sources. Electricity tends to be exceedingly scarce in Casablanca's Shantytowns. Hence, many households must resort to illegally tapping electricity from surrounding electrical networks. The negative health consequences of such illegal connections are far-reaching, and often include accidents resulting in fatalities.

## Sanitation in Tunis, Tunisia

The discussion in this section begins with an examination of the hygiene and sanitation issues confronting Tunisia as a nation. This is necessary to contextualize the subsequent more focused analysis of the issues as they play out in Tunis, the nation's capital city. Tunisia stands out as the country with the most extensive water and sanitation coverage in Northern Africa. The coverage for improved water is nearly 100 per cent in urban areas and nearly 90 per cent in rural areas (WHO/ UNICEF, 2010). Table 8.5 shows that sanitation conditions have been steadily improving in the country since 1990. As the table shows, access to improved sanitation increased from 95 to 96 per cent between 1990 and 2008. The proportion of those depending on shared sanitation facilities has always been low at two per cent. Also worthy of note is the fact that the proportion of the urban population practicing open defecation in the country decreased from 3 per cent in 1995 to non-existent since 2005. However, as Table 8.6 shows, levels of open defecation remain high in rural areas even though they have been steadily declining. A rather paradoxical trend depicted on Table 8.6 has to do with the proportion of the rural population using unimproved sanitation facilities. As the table shows, rather than decline, this proportion has been increasing. It rose from four per cent in 1990 to 14 per cent since 2005 through 2008. A possible explanation for this anomaly is as follows. Commensurate with the recent surge in the population has been a growth and proliferation of spontaneous settlements. These settlements are notorious for their poor sanitation conditions. Thus, an increase in the number of such settlements would invariably trigger a corresponding increase in the dependence on unimproved sanitation facilities.

**Table 8.5 The use of improved sanitation facilities in urban Tunisia,
        1990–2008**

| Year | Facility for Human Waste Disposal | | | |
|------|-------------------|---------------|---------------------|------------------------|
|      | Improved (%) | Shared (%) | Unimproved (%) | Open Defecation (%) |
| 1990 | 95 | 2 | 0 | 3 |
| 1995 | 95 | 2 | 1 | 2 |
| 2000 | 95 | 2 | 2 | 1 |
| 2005 | 96 | 2 | 2 | 0 |
| 2008 | 96 | 2 | 2 | 0 |

*Source*: WHO/UNICEF (2010).

**Table 8.6 Access to improved sanitation facilities in rural Tunisia, 1990–2008**

| Year | Facility for Human Waste Disposal | | | |
|------|-------------------|----------------|-------------------|----------------------|
|      | Improved (%)      | Shared (%)     | Unimproved (%)    | Open defecation (%)  |
| 1990 | 44                | 6              | 4                 | 46                   |
| 1995 | 51                | 6              | 7                 | 36                   |
| 2000 | 57                | 7              | 11                | 25                   |
| 2005 | 64                | 8              | 14                | 14                   |
| 2008 | 64                | 8              | 14                | 14                   |

*Source*: WHO/UNICEF (2010).

More than half of the households in the country have in-house flush toilets. The toilet and cognate facilities are connected to an extensive sewerage network. The rate of connection to the network increased from 21 per cent to 36 per cent between 1975 and 1987 (Souissi, 2001). This rate skyrocketed to 82 per cent in 2007. Despite the country's laudable record on hygiene and sanitation coverage, it continues to face a number of challenges. One factor that has contributed to compounding the challenges is the fact that the country has experienced increasing levels of urbanization and population growth. This rapid increase is exemplified by the fact that the urbanized population rose from less than 50 per cent (49%) in 1975 to 61 per cent barely two decades later in 1994 (Souissi, 2001). One consequence of the sharp rise in levels of urbanization in Tunisia has been a proliferation of informal settlements. Despite the government's efforts to expand coverage, these settlements remain relatively underserved by hygiene and sanitation facilities. Most of the informal settlements are located on the fringes of the capital city, Tunis. By some estimates, informal settlements cover as much as 32 per cent of the urbanized space in Tunis (Souissi, 2001).

*Hygiene, sanitation and environmental conditions in Tunis*

Tunis has a history that dates back to ancient times. It evolved from part of the great ancient city of Carthage, which was founded in 814 BCE (Larbi and Leitmann, 1994: 292). Carthage served as the capital of the Punic trading empire in ancient times. The building of the *casbah*, which became the heart of the *medina* was undertaken by the Almohades subsequent to the Byzantine conquest (circa, 530 CE). The *medina* is the historic Arabic centre of the city. Accordingly, it has always received the genre of attention reserved for city centres. This attention manifested itself in terms of the concentration of public infrastructure. The status of Tunis was embellished in modern history by French colonial authorities. The city was designated as the administrative capital of Tunisia when it became a French protectorate in the 1880s. This period marked the beginning of modern public infrastructure building in the city. The period also witnessed the emergence of modern or Western-style building codes. The codes prescribed construction standards, especially for the areas that went under the appellation, *villes nouvelles* or new towns. These areas served as exclusive European enclaves. Consequently, they were furnished with sanitation facilities equivalent to what was in vogue in Europe at the time. Initially, septic tanks served as the receptacle for sewage. Later, central sewerage systems were introduced. The colonial sewerage network formed the nucleus around which the city's modern sewage system has been developing. The same holds true for the wastewater treatment system.

The extensive sewage, wastewater and storm drainage system of Tunis notwithstanding, the city faces a number of environmental problems attributable to sanitation. The problems have mainly been a function of one thing. Efforts to extend the sanitation, wastewater, and storm drainage networks of Tunis have not kept pace with its population, industrial and spatial growth. Consequently, waste and stormwater run-off, effluents from polluting industries, uncontrolled dumping of municipal and industrial solid wastes, and chemicals from farmland run-off have posed serious threats to the city's wellbeing (Larbi and Leitmann, 1994). The areas most threatened in this regard are the basins in northern Tunis, especially the Medjerda valley, the source of most of the city's water.

Again, as stated above, Tunis is heads and shoulders above its peers in northern Africa with respect to sanitation coverage. As far back as 1991, 98 per cent of households in the District of Tunis had flush toilets (Larbi and Leitmann, 1994). However, when the entire Tunis metropolitan area is taken into account, the proportion with flush toilets falls by more than half to 40 per cent. In the spontaneous areas the proportion is a lot less at 30 per cent. Contrary to what obtains in sub-Saharan African cities, untreated sewage is seldom released into the environment in Tunis. Rather, the sewage is given secondary treatment prior to being discharged into the Mediterranean Sea. A significant portion of the treated sewage is used for agricultural irrigation purposes.

**Conclusion**

The chapter has portrayed Northern Africa as the only region in Africa on track to meet the hygiene, water and sanitation targets of the Millennium Development Goals (MDGs). Yet, using the MDGs as the gauge for measuring success in hygiene and sanitation may be misleading. To be sure, simply halving the proportion of people without access to improved water and sanitation by 2015 is a very low standard for measuring success in this regard. Such a standard may lead to myopic initiatives that seek to simply increase the stock of sanitation facilities and invariably expand sanitation coverage. Similarly, a narrow view of hygiene may lead to efforts designed to ensure that garbage is collected, thereby keeping human settlements clean. As suggested in the case of Egypt, such a simplistic treatment of hygiene and sanitation problems may have unintended negative consequences. When this occurs we must conclude that the strategy summoned to arrest a hygiene and/or sanitation problem is unsustainable. To be considered effective, a strategy to improve hygiene and sanitation conditions must neither have negative externalities nor create any new problems of its own.

# Chapter 9
# Solid Waste Disposal and Sanitation Technologies, and Determinants of Access to Improved Sanitation

## Introduction

In a way, garbage and sanitation are similar to death. Like death, both issues are inescapable, but unpleasant to discuss. Hardly anyone considers trash and excreta issues that can or should be broached at the dining table. Yet, matters of trash and excreta must be dealt with in one way or another wherever there is human activity. People have always been preoccupied with questions of solid and human wastes since the genesis of human settlements. Therefore, there is hardly a society in existence without its own indigenous technology or system of handling garbage and faecal matter. However, it is erroneous to assume that all garbage and/or excreta disposal technologies and systems are environmentally, economically and socio-culturally sustainable. Clearly, some technologies and systems fair better than others from a sustainability perspective. However, the dearth of knowledge on this subject has deprived interested parties of the opportunity to compare and contrast these technologies.

One objective of this chapter is to contribute to efforts to promote knowledge of the various garbage handling systems, and sanitation technologies in use in Africa. Knowledge of these technologies constitutes a logical starting point for any meaningful attempt to adopt sustainable strategies for garbage and excreta management. The need to entertain questions of sustainability is heightened in the case of African countries for many obvious reasons. For instance, there is the issue of cultural differences between these countries and the European nations that colonized them. Yet, as discussed in previous chapters, there has always been a tendency to transfer technology verbatim from Europe or some other Western locale to Africa. Also, there are significant geographic, socio-economic and cultural differences among different regions of the continent. Thus, a technology from one region must be carefully examined before it can be adopted in another.

Another objective of the chapter is to identify some major determinants of accessibility to improved sanitation facilities on the continent. An understanding of factors influencing accessibility to improved sanitation is essential as an input to the hygiene and sanitation policy making process. Such an understanding is also necessary for scholarly research on hygiene and sanitation in Africa. As previous chapters have suggested, access to sanitation is by far greater in Northern Africa than in other regions of the continent. Clearly, therefore, interregional differences exist with respect to access to sanitation facilities. The differences are also present at the international and intra-national levels. Thus, access to sanitation is greater in some countries than in others. Similarly, some towns and cities enjoy better access to sanitation than others within the same country. What factors account for these differences? This question is dealt with later in the chapter.

**Garbage disposal systems**

The volume of urban solid waste in Africa has surged in recent decades thanks to rapid population growth rates and hyper-urbanization trends. The district of Tunis in Tunisia's capital city for instance, was already generating 1,600 tons of solid waste daily in the 1990s (Larbi and Leitman, 1994: 95). About a quarter of this (25–30%) was industrial and commercial waste while the rest was of the domestic genre. It is necessary to note that the garbage collection and disposal system of Tunis is well-organized. By African standards, this is an exception and certainly not the norm. In most parts of the continent, littering or the indiscriminate disposal of garbage is commonplace. Before delving further into the nature of littering, it is necessary to identify the different methods of garbage disposal in use on the continent. The most commonly used of these methods are as follows (Njoh, 2003: 173):

- Littering;
- Open dumps;
- Sanitary landfills;
- Incineration;
- Composting; and
- Disposing of thrash in recovery plants.

*Littering*

Littering is the indiscriminate disposal of waste. Such disposal can occur on streets, along highways, bodies of moving or standing water such as rivers or lakes. In some cases, this may be behind residential units. This is especially the case in informal settlements or slums. Figure 9.1 is illustrative of this latter instance. Note that the garbage in the photograph is comprised mainly of non-bio-degradable material such as plastic. Thus, apart from being simply repugnant and abhorrent, littering poses a serious danger to the environment. For this reason, there are laws, albeit, seldom enforced, against littering in every country in Africa. Gambia, for instance has what it calls anti-littering laws in force (Ceesay, 2009). In South Africa there are by-laws specifically dealing with littering. For instance, the first of Johannesburg's two-part inner-city enforcement strategy deals with a number of violations, including littering, and illegal dumping (Memeza, Online).[1] As these examples suggest, the problem is not that there are no laws against littering. Rather, evidence points to other reasons for the perpetual problem of littering in Africa. Prominent in this regard is the fact that littering by-laws are almost never enforced. Consider the case of Cameroon (Njoh, 2003). Here, the country's copious penal code has provisions for penalizing littering. These provisions have existed for more than four decades. As noted in a Cameroon Tribune article of September 16, 1999, anti-littering legislation had been promulgated since 1967. As stipulated in Section R. 367 of the law, littering and/or failure to participate in street cleaning are punishable by a fine of up 1,200 francs (i.e., about US$2.50 by the current exchange rate of US$1.00 = 486 frs CFA). However, law enforcement authorities never bother to enforce this law.

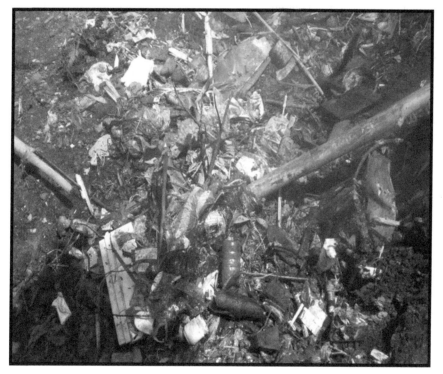

**Figure 9.1 On-site littering**
*Source*: Author's personal photo library.

---

1 This first part falls under the "streets group." The second part, known as the 'Buildings' group, covers building codes. Particularly, it focuses on buildings which have been designated as problematic. This may be because they are suffering from physical obsolescence or are overcrowded. As noted at the outset of this book, this issue is of centrality in the discourse on urban planning as an instrument of public health.

*Open dumps*

This appellation is derived from the fact that the specific locale used for disposing (or dumping) waste is neither enclosed nor covered. The origins of open dumps as a waste disposal strategy can be traced to the United States of the early-1900s (Pitchel, 2005; Blumberg and Gotlieb, 1989). Open dumps grew and proliferated in the US for one main reason. Vast tracts of inexpensive land 'suitable' for dumping were available at the outskirts of the growing cities and suburbs of the 1940s. Initially, dumping consisted simply of direct disposal of garbage on a selected parcel of land, followed by abandonment of that parcel (Pitchel, 2005). Typically selected for this purpose were wetlands, which at the time were considered a 'nuisance.' Although dumping has almost been completely abandoned in the US, it continues to be the strategy of choice in Africa. Here, the dominant method is that of dumping and subsequent abandonment of the land. Thus, by African standards, an open dump is simply an open field designated as a site for the 'dumping' of solid and/or liquid waste. While the sites may serve as a source of valuable recyclable material for scavengers, they can be criticized on many grounds. First, such sites are unsightly and constitute an eye sore. Second, they serve as breeding ground for rats, flies, and vermin. Third, they pose potential hazards such as wildfire. Fourth, they emit pungent odours and can be environmentally hazardous. In this latter regard, open dumps can render otherwise fertile soil barren. This is because the garbage disposed of at such locales usually contains non-degradable materials such as plastics.

*Sanitary landfills*

Sanitary landfills constitute a vast improvement over open dumps. A typical landfill consists of an excavated piece of land into which garbage is dumped and then covered with a layer of earth once it is full. The excavation and soil layer that covers the excavated pit ensure that landfills are not as unsightly as open dumps. However, landfills tend to have the same negative environmental consequences as open dumps. For instance, they constitute a significant threat to groundwater through surface run-off and leaching. There have been some efforts to improve sanitary landfills. Resulting from these efforts is what can be called modified landfills. The modification process entails covering the landfill with a fresh layer of soil, and compacting same every day. The compaction and frequent covering with fresh soil ensures a significant reduction in problems associated with aesthetics, disease, pests, air and water pollution.

*Incineration*

Solid waste incineration is rooted in indigenous African ethos. In ancient times it was commonplace for domestic garbage to be disposed of by burning. However, incineration as a waste disposal strategy in contemporary Africa owes its origins to European colonialism. Two groups of European powers, the British and the Germans, who were active in the colonization of Africa, were also instrumental in developing modern incineration technology. The first modern solid waste incinerator system was developed by the British (Pitchel, 2005). This incinerator went into operation in Nottingham in 1874. About two decades later, a similar incinerator was developed in Germany. In 1882, a cholera outbreak wreaked havoc on Hamburg causing other cities to deny it garbage dumping privileges. Consequently, municipal authorities in Hamburg were forced to seek alternative means of handling the city's ever-growing volume of garbage. In one instance, the authorities turned to British engineers for technical advice. With the assistance of these engineers, authorities in Hamburg succeeded in building Germany's first solid waste incinerator. To be sure, this system is technologically sophisticated. As such, it requires expensive equipment, skilled operators and regular maintenance. Apart from this, the system poses several environmental problems. For instance, fly ash from the incinerator can cause significant damage to air quality.

*Composting*

This waste disposal strategy is also rooted in indigenous African ethos. It is suitable for organic waste, and emerges as the most environmentally friendly of all the waste disposal systems discussed thus far. It involves the careful disposal of organic waste such as food and plant matter in a manner that facilitates their biological decomposition. It is very simple in that biological decomposition of organic waste requires very little more than controlled aerobic conditions. Under these conditions, which simply require oxygen, organic waste is decomposed by bacteria, fungi, worms and a combination of other organisms. The method is environmentally advantageous because of its tremendous ability to enrich the soil. In this regard, it is not only environmentally sustainable but also economically viable. This is especially because the system reduces or even eliminates the need for artificial fertilizers.

**Table 9.1 Comparison of alternative waste disposal systems**

| Method | Merits | Demerits |
|---|---|---|
| Littering | Easy | Unsightly; expensive to clean up; wasteful |
| Open | Easy to manage; low initial investment and operating costs; can be put into operation in a short time. | Unsightly; breeds disease-carrying pests; foul odours; causes air pollution when waste matter is burnt; can contaminate groundwater through leaching, and runoff; can damage ecological valuable marshes and wetlands. |
| Sanitary landfill | Easy to manage; relatively low initial investment costs; can be put into operation in a short time; if properly designed and operated, minimizes pest, aesthetic problems, disease and air and water pollution problems; methane gas produced by waste decomposition can be used as fuel; can receive all kinds of energy; waste can be used to reclaim and enhance the value of sub-marginal land. | Can degenerate into an open dump if not properly designed and managed; requires large amount of land; difficult to find sites because of rising land cost; wasteful use of resources; leaching; may cause water pollution; methane gas from de-composting waste can create fire or explosion hazard; obtaining adequate cover material may be difficult; hauling waste to distant sites is costly and wasteful. |
| Incinerator | Removes odours and disease-carrying organic matter; reduces volume of waste by at least 80%; extends life of landfills; requires little land; can produce income from salvage metals and glass and use of waste heat for domestic purposes. | High initial investment; high operating costs; frequent and costly maintenance and repairs; requires skilled operators; resulting residue and fly ash must be disposed of; causes air pollution unless very costly controls are installed; fine particle-air pollution. |
| Composting | Converts organic waste to soil conditioner that can be sold for use on land; moderate operating costs; most diseases-causing bacteria are destroyed. | Can be used only for organic waste; waste must be separated; limited market as most people are not aware of the use of soil conditioner. |

| Method | Merits | Demerits |
|---|---|---|
| Resource Recovery | High public acceptance; produces air and water pollutants; reduces waste of resources; extends life of landfill; can provide a source of income for people in the informal sector; can be a source of domestic energy; may be easier to find site than for landfill. | High initial investment; high operating costs; technology for many operations not fully proven; requires markets for recovered materials or energy produced; costly maintenance and repairs; requires skilled operators; can cause air pollution if not properly controlled; profitable only with high volume waste; discourages low technology and therefore unsustainable in resource-scarce settings. |

*Source*: Njoh (2003: 175–176).

*Resource recovery*

This is yet another technologically complex waste disposal strategy. Recovery plants are usually large mechanical equipment designed to segregate solid waste based on attributes such as 'degree of solidity.' Their ability to effectuate such segregation means they can separate metal from non-metal wastes. Therefore, they can serve as a preliminary process in an environmentally conscious waste management system. Such plants offer other benefits, including but not limited to, the ability to convert waste into electrical energy. Their advantages notwithstanding, resource recovery plants have very little chance of success in African countries. For one thing, as stated above, they are technologically complicated. For another thing, they require a prohibitively high initial capital outlay. Thus, employing such technology would require dependence not only on foreign financial support but also foreign expertise.

## Conceptualizing sanitation

To meaningfully compare sanitation technologies especially in terms of their effectiveness, it is necessary to begin by clarifying the concept of sanitation. Sanitation has been defined as "the means of collecting and disposing of excreta and community liquid waste in a hygienic way so as not to endanger the health of individuals or the community as a whole" (Cotton et al., 1995: 6). It has also been defined to include "the safe and sound handling (hygiene) and disposal of human excreta including people's approach to satisfy their primal urge" (Freiberger, 2007: 7, quoting Avvannavar and Mani, 2007). The common theme in both definitions is the issue of collection and disposing of human waste. Three major activities are therefore of relevance to a sanitation system. The first is collection, while transportation and treatment (both imbibed within the notion of 'disposing') constitute the second and third respectively. Before delving further into this line of thinking, it is necessary to examine the factors that affect or can affect an individual's approach to, or choice of sanitation facilities. These factors are associated with four major substantive areas, namely human settlements, natural environment, religion and culture, society (Avvannavar, 2007, cited in Freiberger, 2007). Imbibed within the folds of the first factor are, human settlement attributes such as density, the natural setting and the urban natural environment. These factors have implications for the availability of space for sanitation. By extension, therefore, the factors affect people's feelings. These may be feelings about, and view of, habits such as the preference for open defecation or indoor toilets, or the sharing of sanitation facilities with persons of the opposite sex. Natural environmental factors include vegetation, terrain, climatic conditions and the availability of water. Some or all of these factors affect in one way or another, the functioning of flush toilets, sewers or open defecation. Religion and culture are inextricably intertwined and significantly impact people's view of excreta. In some cases, they may be rituals associated with the act of defecating. In essence, how excreta is perceived and related to can have far-reaching implications for the use of different sanitation technologies.

## Sanitation technologies in comparative perspectives

The literature contains descriptions for many sanitation technologies. Analysts have proffered different ways for categorizing the alternative strategies. Elisabeth Freiberger proposes a classification scheme, which borrows generously from Ujang and Henze (2006). Her method groups the technologies on the basis of the three major phases of human and domestic waste management, including collection, transportation and treatment. To be sure, some systems contain only one of these phases while others roll the collection and treatment phases into one. Systems of the latter genre, are apropos for rural and peri-urban settings. These systems have been copiously described by Morgan (2007). Morgan describes one method for collecting and treating human excreta that needs to be briefly discussed before examining improved sanitation facilities. It is the simple dig-and-cover or 'cat method.' It involves simply digging a hole in the ground, defecating in it, and then covering the excreta with soil. Characterizing it as a slightly upgraded version of open defecation, Morgan contends that the method is environmentally friendly. This is because it permits excreta to quickly decompose into compost since it is surrounded by soil. However, the method has many drawbacks. For one thing, it has limited application as it can be used only where there is a vast amount of unused land, and where the soil is loose. In the context of this book, the method does not qualify as a form of improved sanitation.

**Low-cost improved sanitation technologies**

By far the most common sanitation technology for collecting human waste is the pit latrine. There are several variations of the pit latrine. A rather relaxed categorization schema includes the following five varieties (Freiberger, 2007; Morgan, 2006; Ujang and Henze, 2006; Cotton et al., 1995):

- Traditional pit latrine;
- Pit latrine with concrete slab and cover;
- Shallow pit compost latrine;
- Shallow double pit compost latrine; and
- Ventilated improved pit (VIP) latrines.

*The traditional pit latrine*

As stated above, this is by far the most common technology for collecting human waste throughout Africa. The traditional pit latrine comprises three major components as follows. A pit dug into the ground, a platform of wood, earth or concrete slab fitted with a squatting hole, and the superstructure or latrine house (enclosing the platform). The traditional pit latrine has many advantages. It is easy to construct and inexpensive. However, it is saddled with a number of problems. First, it is notorious for releasing pungent odours, and is fly-ridden (especially during the hotter months). Second, pit latrines of the wooden platform variety are vulnerable to termite action, and can easily collapse. Third, they can be challenging to develop in areas with either very unstable or rocky soil. The photograph designated as Figure 9.2 shows how challenging it can be to dig a pit in unstable soil.

Pit latrines tend to lose some of their relative advantage as an inexpensive sanitation technology in such soils. This is because of the extra cost involved in lining and reinforcing the walls of the pit to prevent them from collapsing. Figure 9.3 reflects some of the extra effort necessary to reinforce the pit in unstable soil.

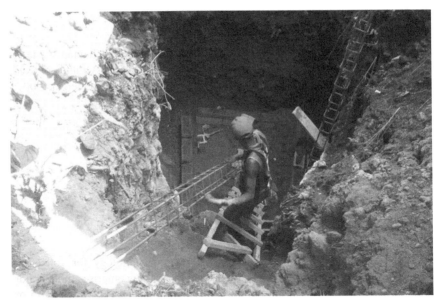

**Figure 9.2 Difficulties digging hole for pit latrine in unstable soil**

*Source*: Photographed by author during fieldwork in Cameroon.

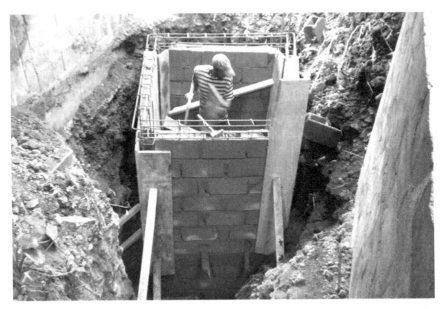

**Figure 9.3 Lining and reinforcement of hole walls required for pit latrines in unstable soil**

*Source*: Photographed by author during fieldwork in Cameroon.

*Pit latrine with concrete slab and cover*

This is simply a slightly improved version of the traditional pit latrine. The improvement consists of fitting the wooden or earth platform with a concrete slab. The concrete slab is then fitted with handles to facilitate portability. In addition, it is fitted with a squatting hole. With a concrete slab and cover, the latrine is more hygienic and easier to clean than latrines of the traditional variety.

*Shallow pit compost latrine*

This system is comprised of a shallow (no deeper than 1 meter) unlined pit. A removable concrete slab is used to cover the pit. This slab serves as the platform on which ash and soil are mixed for use as compost matter. The ash and soil combine to improve the soil's fertility. The ash also serves to reduce odours and flies. It is usually removed once the pit is two-thirds full. The pit serves a composting function in efforts to grow trees, and vegetables. The excreta works well to fertilize the soil, thereby facilitating the growth of plants. Spreading ash on latrine floors as a means of limiting the emission of odours and deterring flies is part of the indigenous ethos in many parts of Africa. The use of ash as a soil nutrient is also indigenous to Africa.

*Shallow double pit latrine*

As the name suggests, this sanitation system is comprised of two composting pits. The pits are usually 1.5 meters deep (Morgan, 2007). These pits may be contained within a permanent structure or portable structure. Soil and ash are regularly added to accelerate composting. As Morgan (2007) noted, the system functions on a 12-month cycle. This allows sufficient time for backfilling the pit and for the excreta to decompose and become fertile for plant life. The compost is usually removed from one pit for the slab to be moved from the filled pit to an empty one. The filled pit is then covered with a thick layer of soil. Trees or vegetables can then be planted directly on the backfilled soil to make direct use of the faeces as manure.

*The ventilated improved pit (VIP) latrine*

The VIP latrine is, as the appellation intimates, a vastly improved version of the traditional pit latrine. It has the advantage of reducing or eliminating odours and flies. It includes one or more vent pipes. These pipes help to conduct odours from the pit to a point above the roof of the latrine house (see Figure 9.4). The sketch shown in the figure is of a VIP latrine with one vent. Apart from conducting odours, the vent also serves as a fly trap. The VIP latrine functions in the following manner (Freiberger, 2007: 8).

An air flow is created by the wind outside the vent pipe. The flow sucks the fetid air out of the latrine … Proper construction means a dark inside of the superstructure to encourage flies to leave the toilet through the vent pipe and a fly screen at the top end of the vent pipe.

Like traditional pit latrines, VIP latrines are extolled for their simplicity, ease of construction and inexpensive cost. However, as the photograph labeled as Figure 9.5 shows, these advantages do not hold under strict scrutiny. Notice that all the construction materials employed in the project depicted in the photograph have a high input of imported materials. For instance, the blocks and concrete contain cement that is manufactured with a high dose of imported ingredients. The concrete reinforcement rods are all imported. The three pipes used to ventilate the pit are also imported.

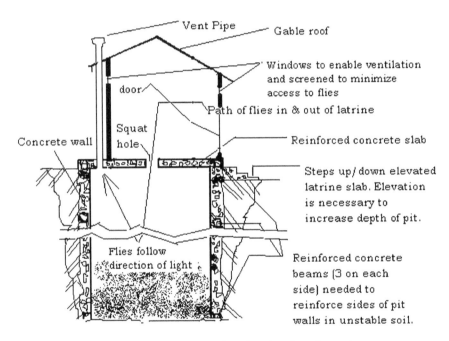

**Figure 9.4 Cross-section of a VIP latrine showing how it works**

*Source*: Author's sketch (not to scale).

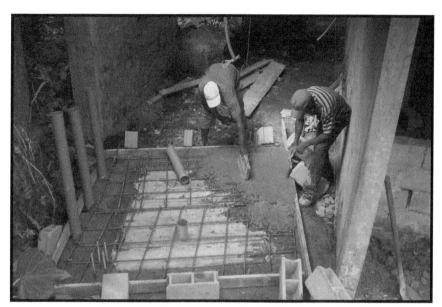

**Figure 9.5 Casting a slab in-situ on a ventilated improved pit latrine pit**
*Source*: Photographed by author during fieldwork in Cameroon.

An increasingly common sanitation technology in Africa is the flush toilet. This technology was originally introduced in Africa by colonial authorities. A variation of this technology is the pour-flush toilet. Given its rising popularity on the continent, the flush toilet is discussed in greater detail below.

*Flush toilet*

The flush toilet is the sanitation system of choice and a mark of modernization for middle- and upper-income households in Africa. It uses water to flush excreta away for storage, transportation and treatment (Freiberger, 2007). The system is the most hygienic of all existing sanitation systems in Africa. However, it has two major drawbacks. The first is its cost. This cost is prohibitively high for the poor. The second is its heavy dependence on water. This can be a serious problem in areas with limited access to water. It is also less functional in most cities of the developing world, especially where water services are frequently interrupted. Thus, flush toilets tend to be used as pour-flush systems in most African cities.

**Factors affecting accessibility to improved sanitation in Africa[2]**

Given the importance of water for hygiene and sanitation, we would be remiss if we did not say a thing or two about Africa's water situation. Africa manifests extremities when it comes to the availability of water. On the one hand, the continent is blessed with abundant water resources. In this regard, the continent is home to large rivers such as the Congo, Nile, Zambezi and Niger, as well as large lakes such as Lake Victoria-Nyanza, the world's second largest fresh water lake. At the same time, the continent is the world's driest. It is surpassed in this regard only by Australia (WWF, Online). Thus, while some parts of the continent enjoy an abundance of water, other areas face severe water shortages, throughout the year. Thus, as Table 9.2 shows, water, like other natural resources, is unevenly distributed across the continent. Some African countries count amongst the nations most endowed with water resources. Others find themselves among the most deprived in this connection. For instance, as Table 9.2 reveals, two African countries, Gabon and Congo (PR) are among the top ten nations of the world with respect to the availability of natural water. Congo occupies the seventh position, and boasts a total of 275 thousand cubic meters of water per capita per year (275,679 m3/cap./year). On its part, Gabon ranks 9 out 180 countries in the world, in this regard. The country boasts 133 thousand cubic meters per capita per year (133,333 m3/capita/year). Table 9.3 highlights the continent's water problem as one largely pertaining to distribution. Some areas have too much water for too few people, while other parts have too little water for too many people. For instance, as the World Wildlife Foundation has noted, the Congo basin into which 30 per cent of Africa's water drains contains only 10 per cent of the continent's population (WWF, Online, para. 1).

---

2    The material in this section has been culled directly from my article in Cities (see Njoh and Akiwumi, 2011).

## Table 9.2 Water availability in Africa in international perspectives

| Item | Country | International Rank | Water Resources [Total Resources: Total Renewable Per Capita (M³/ Capita/Year)] |
|------|---------|-------------------|-----------------------------------------------------------------------|
| 01. | Congo | 7 | 275,679 |
| 02. | Gabon | 9 | 133,333 |
| 03. | Liberia | 15 | 79,643 |
| 04. | Equatorial Guinea | 21 | 56,893 |
| 05. | Central African Republic | 28 | 38,849 |
| 06. | Sierra Leone | 31 | 36,322 |
| 07. | Guinea | 36 | 27,716 |
| 08. | Guinea Bissau | 39 | 25,855 |
| 09. | Congo (DR) | 41 | 25,183 |
| 10. | Madagascar | 46 | 21,102 |
| 11. | Cameroon | 49 | 19,192 |
| 12. | Sao Tome & Principe | 51 | 15,797 |
| 13. | Angola | 55 | 14,009 |
| 14. | Mozambique | 61 | 11,814 |
| 15. | Namibia | 65 | 10,211 |
| 16. | Zambia | 66 | 10,095 |
| 17. | Botswana | 71 | 9,345 |
| 18. | Mali | 75 | 8,810 |
| 19. | Gambia | 87 | 6,332 |
| 20. | Chad | 90 | 5,453 |
| 21. | Cote d'Ivoire | 92 | 5,058 |
| 22. | Swaziland | 93 | 4,876 |
| 23. | Mauritania | 95 | 4,278 |
| 24. | Senegal | 96 | 4,182 |
| 25. | Benin | 99 | 3,954 |
| 26. | Togo | 109 | 3,247 |
| 27. | Niger | 111 | 3,107 |
| 28. | Uganda | 115 | 2,833 |
| 29. | Ghana | 119 | 2,756 |
| 30. | Tanzania | 124 | 2,514 |

| Item | Country | International Rank | Water Resources [Total Resources: Total Renewable Per Capita (M³/ Capita/Year)] |
|------|---------|-------------------|-----------------------------------------------------------------------------------|
| 31. | Nigeria | 125 | 2,514 |
| 32. | Sudan | 129 | 2,074 |
| 33. | Ethiopia | 137 | 1,749 |
| 34. | Eritrea | 139 | 1,722 |
| 35. | Comoros | 140 | 1,700 |
| 36. | Zimbabwe | 143 | 1,584 |
| 37. | Somalia | 144 | 1,538 |
| 38. | Malawi | 145 | 1,528 |
| 39. | Lesotho | 147 | 1,485 |
| 40. | South Africa | 150 | 1,154 |
| 41. | Burkina Faso | 152 | 1,084 |
| 42. | Kenya | 154 | 985 |
| 43. | Morocco | 155 | 971 |
| 44. | Egypt | 156 | 859 |
| 45. | Cape Verde | 158 | 703 |
| 46. | Rwanda | 159 | 683 |
| 47. | Burundi | 161 | 566 |
| 48. | Tunisia | 162 | 482 |
| 49. | Algeria | 163 | 478 |
| 50. | Djibouti | 164 | 475 |
| 51 | Libya | 174 | 113 |

*Source*: WWDR (Online). http://www.unesco.org/bpi/wwdr/WWDR_chart1_eng.pdf.

An analysis of Tables 9.2 and 9.3 also reveals one noteworthy fact. The fact is that the availability of water does not correlate with water accessibility and/or sanitation coverage. For instance, Cape Town, a city in which as many as 96 per cent (95.7%) of its population has access to pipe-borne water, is located in a country, South Africa, which ranks 150th (out of 180) in the world with respect to water availability. More than 90 per cent (90.3%) of the residents of Harare have access to piped water. Yet, Zimbabwe, of which Harare is a part, is ranked 143rd (out of 180 countries) in the world with respect to water availability. Conversely, piped water accessibility is only 15 per cent in Kampala, which is located in Uganda, a country that is ranked 115th in the world with respect to water availability. Thus, factors other than nature account for disparities in water and sanitation coverage in urban areas throughout Africa. What are these factors? Within the context of this book, it is posited that a country's duration as a colony accounts for that country's water and sanitation coverage.

Table 9.3 also contains statistics on water and sanitation accessibility on capital or main cities in selected African countries. As the table shows, accessibility to piped water ranges from a low of 15 per cent for Kampala in Uganda to almost 100 per cent (99.6%) for Cairo, Egypt. The statistics are worse for access to improved sanitation facilities. These statistics range from one per cent for Khartoum, Sudan to about 95 per cent (94.5%) for Harare, Zimbabwe. A closer look at the water and sanitation situation for these two cities, Khartoum and Harare is revelatory.

Khartoum is a large-size African city, with a population of 5.7 million (CIA, Online). Rivers and boreholes (acquifer of about 90–150m deep) serve as the main source of water for this city (UN-Habitat, 2009). The city, like many African cities, suffers from serious water and sanitation problems. Efforts to deal with the problem of water supply in this city include pumping water from boreholes to tanks placed on elevated platforms. The tanks in turn serve as the source of water for domestic use through public standpipes, and private home connections. Residents of poor neighbourhoods typically depend on water vendours for water. Khartoum has no water treatment plant although there is an ongoing project to build one (Biwater, 2010). When completed, the plant will be capable of treating 120,000 $m^3$/day (Ibid).

As is the case in most cities throughout Africa, sanitation, especially the disposal of human waste, is largely a private matter in Khartoum. To be sure, Khartoum has no public toilets. However, in contrast to most cities on the continent, the city has a sewerage network. This network is however small, and serves only 28 per cent of the population. Thus, many households depend on private septic tanks to dispose of human waste. Others, at the urban fringes or peri-urban areas, resort to unhygienic methods of waste disposal, such as shallow pit latrines that facilitate the discharge of raw faecal waste directly into the environment.

**Table 9.3 Water and sanitation situation in selected main or capital cities in Africa, 2003**

| Item | Country | Main or capital city | Per cent with access to piped water | Per cent with access to sewerage | Per cent with access to electricity |
|------|---------|----------------------|-------------------------------------|----------------------------------|-------------------------------------|
| 01. | Angola | Luanda | 13.1 | 20.4 | 36.2 |
| 02. | Benin | Porto Novo | 59.5 | 11.7 | 69.6 |
| 03. | Burkina Faso | Ouagadougou | 33.8 | 12.7 | 54.1 |
| 05. | Cameroon | Yaounde | 33.5 | 26.4 | 98.2 |
| 06. | Cote d'Ivoire | Abidjan | 76.7 | 41.2 | 91.4 |
| 07. | Congo (DR) | Kinshasa | 64.0 | 6.7 | n/a |
| 08. | Egypt | Cairo | 99.6 | 71.9 | 99.8 |
| 09. | Ethiopia | Addis Ababa | 60.8 | 4.2 | 97.1 |
| 10. | Gambia | Banjul | 45.4 | 30.5 | n/a |
| 11. | Ghana | Accra | 55.5 | 36.6 | 86.4 |
| 12. | Guinea | Conakry | 39.2 | 11.2 | 71.4 |
| 13. | Lesotho | Maseru | 42.0 | 5.5 | 18.1 |
| 14. | Mali | Bamako | 49.0 | 30.2 | 64.6 |
| 15. | Morocco | Casablanca | 83.1 | 87.6 | 96.1 |
| 16. | Mozambique | Maputo | 65.4 | 22.1 | 39.2 |
| 17. | Nigeria | Lagos | n/a | n/a | 99.8 |
| 18. | Rwanda | Kigali | 35.1 | 2.8 | 47.5 |
| 19. | South Africa | Cape Town | 95.7 | 93.8 | 92.0 |
| 20. | Sudan | Khartoum | n/a | 1.0 | 54.2 |
| 21. | Uganda | Kampala | 15.1 | 13.6 | 57.1 |
| 22. | Tanzania | Dar es Salaam | 62.0 | 4.4 | 57.7 |
| 23. | Zambia | Ndola | 67.3 | 72.7 | 53.0 |
| 24. | Zimbabwe | Harare | 90.3 | 94.5 | 87.8 |

*Source*: Compiled from UN-Habitat (2009).

On the other extreme of the water and sanitation spectrum in Africa is Harare in Zimbabwe. As Table 9.3 shows, most residents of Harare have access to piped water and improved sanitation facilities. A large proportion of the city's population, particularly within the recognized residential districts has flush toilets (UNEP/IETC, 2002). In addition, it is worth noting that flush toilets in Harare are not limited to upper- and medium-income families. Rather, some of the beneficiaries of these sanitation facilities include low-income families. Harare is also unusual in the African context because it boasts an extensive sewerage network. By some estimates, as much as 80 per cent (1.8 million) of the city's population is served by this network (Nhapi et al., 2006). In the context of the central hypotheses of the study discussed here, it is no coincidence that Zimbabwe is one of the countries with the longest colonial experience in Africa. However, the sewerage system in Harare, the country's capital city, is reported to be growing increasingly dysfunctional with negative trends in the country's economy. Most households in the informal settlements depend on pit latrines to dispose of human waste. In addition, some in these settlements openly defecate and directly dispose of other waste into the environment.

As intimated above, the sanitation problems in urban Zimbabwe pale in significance when compared with the situation in most African countries. For instance, in a study of sanitation conditions in informal settlements and low-income districts in Yaounde, the capital city of Cameroon, Bemmo and colleagues (1998) made the following observations. Low-quality latrines, including stilt latrines over ditches or bodies of flowing or still water as well as vacant lots are used for the purpose of disposing of human waste. In other districts septic tanks and improved latrines serve the same purpose. However, the septic tanks and pit latrines, which are used for the disposal of excrement and grey water, are often located near drinking water wells and typically drained into open drainage ditches. More worthy of note is the fact that Yaounde, like most African cities does not have a sewerage network.

## Determinants of water and sanitation deprivation

Throughout the initial chapters of this book, colonialism was identified as the source of many of the hygiene and sanitation problems in African countries. Certainly, access to water and sanitation in Africa cannot be completely explained by colonialism alone. There are other important factors such as poverty, the lack of political will, and culture that are logical and intuitively appealing as determinants of this phenomenon. It must be recalled that hygiene and sanitation policies and technologies were introduced as part of the European colonial project in Africa. Therefore, it makes sense to consider colonialism as an important determinant of the phenomenon.

Accordingly, it is hypothesized that the duration of colonial periods in African countries correlate with improvements in water and sanitation conditions. In other words, longer colonization periods are likely to result in improved water and sanitation conditions than shorter ones. The basis of this hypothesis is easy to appreciate. Colonial powers strived to make life as convenient as possible for colonial officials and other Europeans in the colonial territories. Hence, with the passage of time, the inventory of facilities such as water and sanitation infrastructure designed to attain this objective grew larger. These pieces of infrastructure were left in place with the demise of colonialism. Thus, it is a reasonable expectation that countries in which the colonial era lasted longer inherited a larger inventory of water and sanitation facilities than their counterparts in which this era was brief. Also, to the extent that colonial powers were guided by different philosophies based on their ideological inclinations, it is safe to posit a link between the identity or nationality of the colonizer and water and sanitation provisioning. These two lines of reasoning provide a basis for the following specific hypotheses:

> *Hypothesis I*: The duration of colonization and the colonizer's identity constitute viable predictors of accessibility to water and sanitation facilities in urban Africa.

> *Hypothesis II*: Urban residents in countries with a longer colonial history have greater access to improved water facilities than their counterparts in countries in which the colonial era was brief.

> *Hypothesis III*: Urban residents in countries with a longer colonial history have greater access to improved sanitation facilities than their counterparts in countries in which the colonial era was brief.

The process of testing these three main hypotheses in earnest begins in the next section with a description of the research methodology, including the data, data sources and analytical techniques employed.

## Methodological issues

*Data and data sources*

The data for this study are of the secondary and quantitative genre. The data, which are for 2008, were obtained from the following sources: 1) the US Central Intelligence Agency (CIA) Factbook (CIA, Online), 2) the 'World Bank Data Online' (World Bank, Online), and 3) national government websites of African countries. The CIA Factbook in combination with national government sites served as the source of data on the colonial experience of African countries. (see CIA, Online). The World Factbook, which is available in hard copy and online, contains reliable and up-to-date data on the geography, people, government, economy, communications, transportation, the military, and international affairs of all sovereign nations in the world. Since 1981, the publication, which used to be released semi-annually, has been published every year. It was first made available online in June 1997.

Through the 'World Bank Data Online,' the World Bank Group makes available to the public free-of-charge, up-to-date statistics on living conditions throughout the world (see data.worldbank.org). The database contains information in Arabic, English, French and Spanish on more than 2,000 indicators, including hundreds dating back about half-a-century. This source provided statistics on access to water, sanitation and electricity for urban Africa. It is important to note that the original source for these statistics is the World Health Organization (WHO) and the United Nations Children's Fund (UNICEF), Joint Measurement Programme (JMP). Efforts to secure the data directly from this source were thwarted by the fact that its Universal Resource Locator (URL) was dead and therefore inaccessible.

*Variables and measurements*

Three variables, one dependent (DV) and two independent (IV) are examined in the study. The DV is an index constructed with statistics on the accessibility of improved water and sanitation facilities respectively. Access to improved sanitation facilities in urban areas within any given country is operationalized in terms of the percentage of urban population in that country with at least access to excreta disposal facilities. As defined by the WHO and UNICEF, these facilities must be capable of effectively preventing human, animal and insect contact with excreta (World Bank, Online; WHO, 2007). In practice, such facilities typically range from simple but protected pit latrines to flush toilets with a sewerage connection.

Water accessibility is operationalized in terms of the percentage of a country's urban population with 'reasonable' access to an adequate amount of water from an improved source. The definition of 'improved water source' proffered by WHO and UNICEF is adopted. According to this definition, an improved water source includes, household connection, public standpipe, borehole, protected well or spring, and rainwater (World Bank, Online). Reasonable access is taken to connote the availability of at least 20 liters of water per person per day within one kilometer of the dwelling unit. Conversely, unimproved water sources include vendors, tanker trucks, and unprotected wells and springs.

The mathematical formulation for the index employed as the DV proceeded as follows. Equal weights are given accessibility to water and sanitation respectively. There is no logical reason for assuming that access to one or the other of these facilities is more important. Accordingly, it is assumed that accessibility to both must add up to unity (i.e., 1). Therefore, accessibility to each of the facilities = 0.50 (or ½). This served as the coefficient by which a country's score (percentage of population with access to water or sanitation) is multiplied. The formula for computing the composite score or Index for ACCESS for any given country can be expressed as follows:

ACCESS =

$$\sum_{i=1}^{2} \frac{1}{N(F_i)}$$

The formula can be stated in its more generic form as follows:

$$\sum_{i=1}^{N} \frac{1}{N(F_i)}$$

Where, N = the different types of facilities (in this case, water and sanitation = 2); $F_i$ = the facility number (in this case, facility #1 = water, and facility #2 = sanitation).

One of the IV's, Colonization, was operationalized in terms of the duration of the colonial era in any given country (YRSCOL). This duration, measured in years, is taken to include the period spanning from when an African country came under the effective control of one or more European colonial powers, to when the country gained political independence. The date on which a territory was granted protectorate status by a colonial power was taken to mark the beginning of effective control of that territory.

The second IV, Colonizer Identity, is operationalized in terms of the nationality of the European power that colonized any given African country. It is treated in the study as a dummy variable, which takes on the value '1' if the colonizer was Britain, and '0' otherwise.

*Analytical techniques*

The computer software programme employed in the study is the Predictive Analytic Soft-Ware (PASW) Version 18. For a long time, this software has gone under the name, SPSS (Statistical Program for Social Science). It is a comprehensive and versatile software for analyzing data. It is arguably the most widely used in the social sciences. The analytic techniques employed include cross-tabulations and the concomitant Chi-Square, as well as the Phi-coefficient in the bivariate context. In the multivariate context, the Ordinary Least Squares (OLS) technique is employed. Although a number of other more sophisticated techniques have come along since the OLS was invented in the late-1700s, it remains very popular for purposes of data fitting and determining relations among variables in social science research. Typically, the aim is to adjust parameters of a model function in a manner that can best fit a data set. The link between the dependent and predictor variables in an OLS model can be summarized in the following mathematical terms:

$$Y = a + \beta_1 x \ldots e$$

Where,

$a$ = the intercept;
$\beta 1$ = the slope;
$x$ = the predictor variables;
$Y$ = the dependent variable;
$e$ = the error term.

The concomitant R-square value—a value that lies between 0 and 1—is used to establish the model's "goodness of fit."

Another 'goodness of fit' test employed in the study is the Chi-Square. This statistic, which is useful in instances involving both qualitative and quantitative variables, is employed to determine the probability of an association between the DV and IV in the study. Essentially, it is used to test the null hypothesis that the DV and IV are independent. It helps to guard against an erroneous rejection of the null hypothesis.

**Main findings**

Table 9.4 summarizes the OLS values for the multiple regression model designed to test Hypothesis I. The hypothesis posits colonial duration as a viable predictor of accessibility to improved water and sanitation facilities. The model linking these variables can be expressed in the following mathematical terms:

ACCESS = 41.956 + 0.322 YRSCOL + 2.420 COLONIZER
t:        (7.140)        (4.500)**        (0.649)
**Sig. at $p < 0.000$; R2: 0.334; F: 11.45 (sig. at $p < 0.000$).

Note that the F-statistic associated with the model of 11.545 is statistically significant at the $p < 0.000$. This suggests a very 'good fit' thus, providing grounds for rejecting the null hypothesis of independence between the independent variable (IV) and dependent variable (DV). The DV is the index combining water and sanitation, while the predictor variables are, the duration of colonial era and colonizer identity. Therefore, as hypothesized, the colonizer's identity (in this case, British versus 'others') and colonization, quantified in terms of the duration of the colonial era, measured in years in any given country are viable predictors of access to improved water and sanitation facilities in that country. The coefficient of multiple determination or adjusted R-square value of 0.34 suggests as follows. The duration of the colonial era in, combined with the identity of the colonizer of, any given African country account for as much as 34 per cent of the variability in the percentage of the urban population with access to improved water and sanitation facilities in that country. However, while the contribution of 'colonial duration' to the model is statistically significant (t-value = 4.500 significant at p < 0.000), that of the colonizer's identity, a dummy variable, is not. Yet, it is important to note that this latter is positively associated with the DV.

**Table 9.4 Multiple regression models with the Water and Sanitation Index (WATERSAN) as Dependent Variable**

| PREDICTOR | B | STD. ERR. | T-STAT |
|-----------|-----|-----------|--------|
| YRSCOL | 0.322 | 0.071 | 4.500** |
| COLPWRID | 2.420 | 3.727 | 0.649 |

**Sig.* at p < 0.000; Adj. $R^2$: 0.34 F: 11.545, significant at p < 0.000. Constant: 41.956 (t = 7.140, sig. at 0.000)

To test the second hypothesis, African countries were divided into two groups, classified respectively as 'Low' and 'High' with respect to the percentage of their urban population having access to improved water facilities. The mean of this percentage for all countries in the study served as the cut-off point. Countries with percentages higher than the mean belonged to the 'High' group while those with percentages lower than the mean were classified as 'Low.' A similar classification scheme was developed for the variable 'Duration of Colonial Era' in which countries with below average years of colonization were classified as 'Short' while those with above average years were classified as 'Long.' Table 9.5 is the 2 x 2 contingency table summarizing the related findings. As the table shows, 27 African countries fell under the category of countries with a 'short' colonial era, while 16 belonged to the category of countries with a 'long' colonial experience. Note that 48 per cent (48.1% or 13 out of 27) of the countries with a 'short' colonial experience are recorded as 'High' with respect to the per cent of their urban population with access to improved water facilities. In comparison, almost 88 per cent (87.5% or 14 out of 16) of the urban population in countries with a 'long' colonial duration have 'high' access to improved water facilities. The Chi-Square value associated with the table is 6.659, and statistically significant at the 0.01 level. The Phi-coefficient, which indicates the strength of association is 0.394. The value for this nonparametric measure is indicative of a medium to strong association between the two variables, duration of colonization and percentage of urban population with access to improved water facilities. More importantly, this finding supports Hypothesis II.

### Table 9.5 Per cent of urban population with access to improved water as a function of duration of colonial era

| | | Duration of colonial era | | Total |
|---|---|---|---|---|
| | | Short | Long | |
| Per cent of Urban Population with Access to Improved Water | Low | 14 (51.9%) | 2 (12.5%) | 16 (37.2%) |
| | High | 13 (48.1%) | 14 (87.5%) | 27 (62.8%) |
| | Total | 27 (100%) | 16 (100%) | 43 (100%) |

Chi-Square: 6.659; DF: 1; Sig. (1-tail): 0.010; Phi: 0.394 (Sig.: 0.010).

### Table 9.6 Per cent of urban population with access to improved sanitation as a function of duration of colonial era

| | | Duration of colonial era | | Total |
|---|---|---|---|---|
| | | Short | Long | |
| Per cent of Urban Population with Access to Improved Sanitation | Low | 18 (69.2%) | 3 (18.8%) | 21 (50.0%) |
| | High | 8 (30.8%) | 13 (81.3%) | 21 (50.0) |
| | Total | 26 (100%) | 16 (100%) | 42 (100%) |

Chi-Square: 10.096; DF: 1; Sig. (1-tail): 0.002; Phi: 0.490 (Sig.: 0.001).

To test the tenability of Hypothesis III, the data are manipulated in the same manner as in the case of Hypothesis II. Table 9.6 shows the Chi-square Analysis of the observed relationship between colonization and access to improved water facilities in urban Africa. A perusal of the table reveals that 26 countries with data on access to improved sanitation in urban areas experienced a 'short' colonial period while 16 had a 'long' colonial experience. Only 31 per cent (30.8% or 8 out of 26) of the countries with a 'short' colonial era appeared in the group of countries in which the urban population enjoys 'high' access to improved sanitation facilities. In comparison, as much as 81 per cent (81.3% or 13 out of 16) of the countries with a 'long' colonial experience enjoy "high" access to the same facilities. Thus, clearly, there is a relationship between colonization and access to improved sanitation facilities in urban Africa. The Chi-Square associated with the table is 10.096, which is statistically significant at the 0.002 level and indicative of a strong association. The Phi-coefficient value of 0.490 is strong, and lends further credence to this assertion.

### Discussion and conclusion

The findings support the hypothesis that colonization constitutes a viable predictor of accessibility to water and sanitation facilities in urban Africa. Colonization is quantified in terms of the number of years any given African country spent as a European colony. Accessibility is operationalized in terms of percentage of urban population with access to the facilities in question. Within the framework of this hypothesis, longer, as opposed to shorter, colonization periods result in increased access to water and sanitation facilities. This hypothesized relationship is logical and intuitively appealing. A well-known objective of the European colonial project was to acculturate and assimilate Africans through so-called modernization projects. More importantly, colonial powers attempted to replicate in Africa, living conditions that prevailed in Europe at the time. The resultant in both cases included the development of modern infrastructure facilities of which water and sanitation are a major element. Initially these amenities were developed in exclusive European enclaves. However, over time, the need to attain other objectives of the colonial project such as 'winning the hearts and minds' of Africans, necessitated the introduction of the amenities in other districts of colonial towns. Where colonial governments were not able to directly develop modern infrastructure, they enacted legislation requiring adherence to modern development standards in the built environment. With the passage of time, the inventory of facilities such as water and sanitation infrastructure developed in line with modern standards grew larger. These pieces of infrastructure, most of which were developed by colonial governments, outlived the colonial era in Africa.

Thus, the following is conceivable. Countries with longer colonial histories inherited more pieces of modern infrastructure, including water and sanitation facilities than their counterparts with shorter ones. Within this frame of thinking the finding that colonizer identity is statistically insignificant appears counter-intuitive at first sight. However, a more rigorous analysis uncovers the following incontestable fact. Despite rhetoric to the contrary, the objectives of the colonial project in Africa were the same for all European colonial powers. Accordingly, European colonial powers, without exception strived to ensure a level of comfort for their citizens stationed in the colonies. This entailed, among other things, developing modern water and sanitation infrastructure commensurate with, or at least approximating what obtained in Europe at the time. It is true, as critics maintain that the aim was never to improve living conditions for Africans. However, there is no denying that upon the demise of colonialism, the infrastructure was essentially bequeathed to the emerging post-colonial governments. To the extent that it takes time to develop public infrastructure, it follows that territories with longer periods of European settlement inherited larger inventories than those in which such settlement was brief.

This finding must not be misconstrued as suggesting a return to colonialism in Africa. Nor should it be viewed as an endorsement or glorification of the colonial era. Rather, the finding suggests that despite its reprehensible nature, colonialism has important lessons for contemporary policy-makers in Africa. In particular, the findings have important lessons for those involved in initiatives designed to increase access to improved water and sanitation facilities on the continent. How were colonial governments which operated on measly budgets able to accomplish the daunting task of infrastructure building in Africa? As stated above, these governments enlisted the free labour input of Africans to realize this feat. If colonial authorities were exceedingly successful in this regard, it is because they were quick to recognize an important attribute of the African ethos. This aspect is the propensity of Africans to indulge in communal work. One analyst was quick to make this observation with respect to Tanganyika (present-day, Tanzania). The analyst noted that communal labour was an integral part of the traditional system of many African tribes that was exploited by colonial governments to implement public works projects (Nye, Jr., 1963: 36).

In fact, national governments and municipal authorities in Africa would do well to, like their colonial predecessors, see African communities not only as service delivery sites but also as sources of labour. Communities throughout the continent have already demonstrated their wherewithal to undertake major water and other public infrastructure building projects through self-help initiatives (Njoh, 2006). National government and municipal authorities in these countries would therefore be well advised to incorporate local communities as active participants, and not simply objects, in the development process.

# Chapter 10
# Sustainable Hygiene and Sanitation Strategies

## Introduction

Public health elements of modern building codes and other town planning regulations constitute a colonial legacy in African countries. The decision to transplant these elements to Africa was not motivated by a genuine concern for the health and welfare of Africans. Rather, it was driven by the need to realize critical ideological, economic and political objectives of the colonial project on the continent. The need to foster the ideology of European racial superiority led to the formulation and implementation of health policies that targeted exclusively European enclaves. Indigenous authorities throughout the continent seemingly failed to recognize the originally intended purpose of the policies, and proceeded to adopt them verbatim.

Evidence emerging from the continent reveals that the policies have woefully failed to address its contemporary health problems. Manifestation of this evidence has assumed manifold forms. Unhygienic and insalubrious conditions characterize human settlements from Cairo to Cape Town, and from Dakar to Mogadishu. We have painted a vivid picture of these conditions in their regional contexts in the preceding chapters. It is not enough to simply articulate these problems and retrace the roots of previous efforts to resolve them. Serious steps must be taken to understand and avoid the pitfalls of these efforts. The narrow focus of colonial hygiene and sanitation policies and the fact that they were transplanted from Europe is certainly one reason for their failure in Africa. Simply put, the policies proved to be unsustainable. This underscores an urgent need to develop more sustainable hygiene and sanitation policies. This final chapter seeks to make a modest contribution to efforts designed to address this need. The chapter begins by rationalizing the need to eradicate hygiene and sanitation problems as a socio-economic development strategy. Then, it sheds light on the concept of sustainability especially in the context of hygiene and sanitation in particular and public health in general. Finally, and before concluding, it proposes a few potentially sustainable strategies for improving hygiene and sanitation conditions in resource-scarce settings.

## Hygiene, sanitation and socio-economic development

Hygiene and sanitation are often treated as an objective of development initiatives. Consequently, their role as engines of development is usually ignored in development discourse and practice. When seen exclusively as objects of development, hygiene and sanitation initiatives tend to be treated in isolation. Yet, unless such initiatives are recognized as necessary inputs into other development undertakings, efforts to promote socio-economic development especially in developing countries are unlikely to succeed.

Hygiene and sanitation conditions affect human development, and by extension, national socio-economic development, in multiple ways. Improved hygiene and sanitation have direct implications for public health by reducing the incidence of infectious and communicable diseases such as diarrhea, dysentery, cholera, typhoid, and tuberculosis. This in turn can result in the reduction of morbidity and mortality. The positive impact of hygiene and sanitation on health can be realized by implementing measures as basic as requiring the provision of pit latrines as a prerequisite for building plan approval. To be sure, building codes and/or town planning regulations throughout Africa, particularly because they were imported from European countries, already contain such requirements. The problem is that authorities never bother to ensure their implementation. Consequently, these authorities squander viable opportunities to promote badly needed national and regional socio-economic development. Yet, as implied above, the link between sanitation and development is intuitively appealing. For instance, improved hygiene and sanitation conditions can, among other things, produce the following desirable outcomes (Scott et al., 2003; Coates, 1999):

- Reduction in levels of poverty;
- Improved public revenue generating ability;
- Higher school attendance rates;
- Reduction in child mortality rates;
- Reduction in maternal mortality;
- Empowerment of women.

*Reduction in levels of poverty*

Improved hygiene and sanitation conditions positively affect economic productivity. Conversely, when these conditions are poor, not only individuals, but the economy in general, is negatively impacted. Diseases such as diarrhea, dysentery and cholera that are directly linked to insalubrious conditions render people incapable of working, attending school or participating in any socio-economically productive activity. In addition, valuable and scarce resources have to be expended in efforts to treat victims of these diseases. Those particularly hurt in such circumstances are the poor, who are the most vulnerable to communicable diseases. This tends to hamper poverty reduction initiatives. Thus, rendered incapable by such diseases, the poor cannot meaningfully participate in activities designed to improve their situation. The link between sanitation and poverty has been eloquently articulated in a recent 'talking points' memo by the UN inter-agency coordinating entity, UN Water (see UN Water, 2009). The memo noted that "investments in basic sanitation can help lift people out of poverty, ill health and early death" (Ibid: 1).

*Improved public revenue generating ability*

The consequences of insalubrious conditions are not limited to individuals. In fact, municipal, national and regional governments can also be victimized by the negative health outcomes of such conditions. For instance, a cholera outbreak in any locality can have devastating consequences for that locality's revenue-earning ability. Not only does such an outbreak render the locality's workforce literally unproductive, it also effectively discourages foreign visitors from the locality. Therefore, it is safe to argue that insalubrious conditions have severe consequences for the foreign earnings of say, a country. This is especially true if the country depends on tourism for its economic survival. One case in point is illustrative (Scott, et al., 2003). In 1991-92, Peru was hit by a cholera epidemic. The country suffered a net loss directly associated with the epidemic of $200 million, approximately one per cent of the country's GDP. Prominent among the areas that made up this amount were lost lives, and decreases in production, exports, and tourism. In fact, as experience has shown, investments in sanitation are capable of protecting tourism revenues, which in some countries account for no less than 10 per cent of the GDP (UN Water, 2009: 2). Empirical evidence suggests that developing countries realize nine United States dollars (US$9.00) worth of benefits for every one dollar (US$1.00) spent on improving sanitation facilities (UN Water, 2009: 2). Ailments resulting from insalubrious and unhygienic conditions stifle efforts to deal with other serious diseases and sicknesses in Africa. In fact, "on any typical day, more than half the hospital beds in Sub-Saharan Africa are occupied by patients suffering from faecal-related diseases" (UN Water, 2009: 1). Consequently, resources that would otherwise be spent on promoting economic development are consumed by efforts to treat preventable diseases.

*Higher school attendance rates*

Improved sanitation conditions have also been tied to levels of school attendance. Thus, children are likely to be motivated to attend school if the school environment is clean than otherwise. For example, a programme designed to improve hygiene and sanitation conditions in Bangladeshi schools resulted in boosting the school attendance rates for girls by 11 per cent (Sen, 2000). Similar gains in school attendance due to improved sanitation have also been registered in India. Here, the provision of toilet facilities for girls significantly increased girls' school enrolment levels. To be sure, improvement in sanitation has the potential of increasing school attendance not only for girls but for school-aged children in general. Some 200 million days of school attendance per year are currently lost due to the lack of sanitation (UN Water, 2009: 3). The loss in days of school attendance here is easy to understand. In Africa for instance, most school-aged children are unable to attend school because they are affected by diseases resulting from insalubrious conditions.

*Reduction in child mortality rates*

The most oft-mentioned link between sanitation and development passes through child mortality. Some 1.7 million deaths per annum worldwide are attributed to insalubrious conditions involving dirty and unsafe drinking water, and the improper disposal of human waste (Scott et al., 2003: 4). Particularly noteworthy for the present purpose is the fact that almost all (90 per cent) of these deaths are of children, and occur in developing countries. Improved hygiene and sanitation conditions can prevent child mortality from diarrhea by over 30 per cent (UN Water, 2009: 1). Thus, the connection between sanitation and health is not only theoretical. Rather, this relationship exists in reality. For instance, efforts to improve hygiene and sanitation conditions in Salvador, Brazil produced a decrease in diarrhea-related deaths by as much as 43 per cent in the poorest areas of the City (UN Water, 2009).

*Reduction in maternal mortality rates*

Unhygienic and insalubrious conditions have also been incriminated as a leading cause of maternal mortality. These conditions significantly increase the infection rate of hookworm, a known contributing factor to anaemia, and other ailments such as tetanus that are linked to maternal mortality (Scott et al., 2003). Unsafe drinking water as well as the lack of basic sanitation facilities such as latrines, are at the root of lethal diseases such as diarrhea that claim more than 2 million lives worldwide annually. Improving these facilities can reduce the global disease burden and go a good way in curbing the incidence of such preventable deaths.

*Women empowerment*

Improved hygiene and sanitation conditions have a direct impact on the health of women, and by extension, women empowerment. This is particularly true in Africa. Here, women and girls are central to necessary life-sustaining activities such as the production, management, and safeguarding of water, and the cleaning and upkeep of the residential facilities and their surroundings. The lack or scarcity of say, water facilities thus increases the domestic burden of women and girls. Where there are no piped water facilities, for instance, women and girls tend to spend much time on long journeys to water sources such as springs, rivers and lakes. The lack of sanitation facilities tends to have even more serious, and sometimes life-threatening, consequences for women and girls. For example, the lack of basic facilities such as latrines often means women have to wait to take advantage of the privacy afforded by night-time darkness to urinate or have a bowel movement. Otherwise, they are compelled to travel for considerable distances to secluded areas to attend to nature's call. Delaying urination or bowel movement for several hours can cause irreversible bladder or intestinal damage. Also, the use of secluded locales for sanitary purposes exposes women to many risks, including mugging and sexual assault. Thus, it is safe to conclude that the lack of improved hygiene and sanitation facilities is antithetical to efforts to empower women.

Apart from their direct impact on the health of women, improved sanitation conditions contribute significantly to national economic development. Consider basic improvements such as providing households and/or communities with latrines or toilets. This improvement alone invariably reduces the distance people must cover to reach where they can relieve themselves. The World Health Organization (WHO) estimates that the time saved in this connection has an annual economic value of more than US$114 billion (UN Water, 2009: 2).

## Sustainability in hygiene and sanitation policymaking

Sustainability or some variant thereof, is arguably the most oft-used term in the lexicon of development at both the international and domestic levels today. But what does the term really mean when used in the context of development? In other words, what is the meaning of sustainable development (SD)? The most frequently quoted definition of this term appears in the Brundtland Report, "Our Common Future" (Brundtland Commission, 1987). The definition appears in the report, which was prepared by the World Commission on Environment and Development (WCED) in 1987, and goes as follows:

> Sustainable development is development that meets the needs of the present without compromising the ability of future generations to meet their own needs.

The essence of addressing the needs of the poor, and the importance of acknowledging the finite nature of natural resources are stressed in the report. In particular, world leaders and agents of development are beseeched to ensure the judicious utilization of the world's finite and rapidly depleting pool of natural resources. For a while, the concept of sustainability was tied to natural resources. However, since the Earth Summit in Rio, Brazil in 1992, the term has made its way into the vocabulary of disparate disciplines. Today, the term tends to mean different things to different people. So, what does it mean for a sanitation system to be sustainable? The following definition by Sustainable Sanitation Alliance (SuSanA) is apropos for the purpose of the present discussion.

A sustainable sanitation system is one that is economically viable, socially acceptable, and technically and institutionally appropriate, and should involve a minimal use of scarce (natural) resources (SSA, 2011: 1).

Thus, sanitation entails much more than toilets alone. In fact, to be sustainable, a sanitation system needs to be more encompassing. It includes more than technical elements. In the specific case of improved sanitation, it encompasses various pieces of a sanitation system, and the manner in which these pieces fit together within a broader contextual environment (SSA, 2011: 2). Most importantly, for a sanitation system to be sustainable, it must be embedded within a wider local context. Within the framework of this line of reasoning, the Sustainable Sanitation Alliance (SuSanA) proposes the following as potentially viable approaches to sustainable sanitation:

- Sanitation system approach;
- Public dialogue or advocacy;
- Social change;
- Capacity development and knowledge exchange;
- Participatory planning;
- Sanitation as a productive process; and
- Innovative financing.

*Sanitation systems approach*

As stated above, sanitation encompasses far more than technology. If it has to be sustainable, it must entertain questions of institutional management, community and individual change. This implies that no sanitation system or programme can register any significant success while it depends on a single technology. To be successful, and in fact, sustainable, as SuSanA suggests, the systems would need to account for the entire waste management chain, from collection, transportation, and treatment, to disposal. Urban planners, health officials and others involved in the hygiene and sanitation sector are wont to commit the grave error of treating sanitation technology as universal artifacts. Yet, sanitation technology, like most technology or knowledge in planning is characterized more by uncertainty than by certainty. A word on the prototype conditions under which urban planning occurs is in order here. These conditions are presented in Figure 10.1. As the figure shows, planning practice typically occurs under one of four different conditions, including the following (Njoh, 1999; Christensen, 1985):

- Known technology, agreed goal (Box A);
- Unknown technology, agreed goal (Box B);
- Known technology, no agreed goal (Box C); and
- Unknown technology, no agreed goal (Box D).

| | | G O A L | |
|---|---|---|---|
| | | **AGREED** | **NOT AGREED** |
| **TECHNOLOGY** | **KNOWN** | A | C |
| | **UNKNOWN** | B | D |

**Figure 10.1 Prototype conditions in characterizing planning practice**
*Source*: Christensen (1985); Njoh (1999).

Planning practitioners often proceed on the basis of the conditions represented by Box A. In other words, they operate under the false assumption that there is a consensual goal and a known technology for attaining this goal. This assumption draws inspiration from orthodox planning principles. These principles are inclined to advance planning as a scientific endeavour, and planning schemes as well-tested and proven solutions to fully understood human problems. Thus, planning schemes and technologies are viewed in the same light as a well-tested and approved vaccine against some well-known disease. Such a vaccine, once invented, can simply be administered in prescribed doses in a pre-specified order to millions worldwide. This has been the case with vaccines for smallpox, chickenpox, and common flues.

Proceeding on the basis that there is consensus with respect to goals, and a known technology for any given problem has had serious negative implications in planning practice. Witness the fact that efforts to employ modernist planning tools to resolve planning problems in Africa, as shown in previous chapters have proven woefully unsuccessful. In the area of sanitation, it is becoming increasingly clear that imported technologies, especially of the Western variety, are, for obvious reasons, unsustainable in Africa. Authorities in Africa are therefore beseeched to make serious efforts to locate sanitation technologies of the more appropriate, more affordable, and therefore, more sustainable variety.

Authorities in the sanitation domain in Africa have to be realistic and recognize the fact that they are operating, in most cases, under the conditions represented by Box B (Figure 10.1). It is clear that hygiene and sanitation conditions throughout the continent are in need of improvement—an agreed goal. However, the means to reach this end, that is, the technology, remains largely unknown. Recognizing this truism will invariably lead to more serious efforts to secure sustainable sanitation technology, in other words, sanitation technology that dovetails neatly into Africa's natural, socio-cultural, and politico-economic environment.

One factor accounting for the woeful failures that have been registered by efforts in the sanitation and other development domains in Africa has to do with the tendency to discount African indigenous knowledge and technology. Yet, as shown later in this chapter, there is a wealth of such knowledge and technology that remains largely untapped but hold enormous promise for efforts to improve hygiene and sanitation conditions on the continent. Thus, the following argument appears tenable. Planners and other authorities in the hygiene and sanitation domain, like their counterparts in other domains in Africa, occasionally operate under conditions such as those represented in Box C (Figure 10.1). In this case, as the box suggests, the technology (that is indigenous knowledge), exists but there is no agreed use (goal) to which it should be put. To harness indigenous knowledge and apply it as necessary in the sanitation domain is to make sanitation systems more sustainable.

To be sure, there are many areas in the sanitation domain that are characterized by uncertainty. Consider the established fact that excreta contain valuable nutrients for plants, and have bio-fuel potential that could be of immeasurable utility for energy and other purposes. Yet, the complexity of actually making good use of excreta means any hasty move in that direction may prove catastrophic. For instance, the imprudent use of partially treated or untreated water from sewerage systems invariably results in food products with raw faecal matter winding up on market shelves. The health consequences of such a gaffe are obvious and need not be regurgitated here. However, what this suggests is that planners and other authorities in the sanitation domain in Africa occasionally operate under conditions characterized by Box D (Figure 10.1)—unknown goals and unknown technology.

*Public dialogue and advocacy*

The notion of sustainability entails much more than an exclusive focus on ends. It involves consideration of the means to these ends. More importantly it involves communicating both means and ends to the real or potential beneficiaries of planning initiatives. To ensure sustainability of planned activities, communication must be bi-directional. It must involve candid exchanges or dialoguing between planners and public authorities on the one hand, and planned project/program beneficiaries on the other. One goal of this process is to ensure that institutional authorities and members of the beneficiary communities recognize their stake in the planned project. Institutional authorities are pivotal in this process. This is because they control the financial and other resources necessary for project implementation. These authorities are also responsible for creating the type of legal and regulatory environment required to make any development project (e.g., sanitation) sustainable. The concept of sustainability here needs to be extended to include the extent to which sanitation policy making is capable of inducing or stimulating economic growth. Here, the sanitation domain must be recognized as an avenue for real or potentially gainful economic activities.

As mentioned earlier, sanitation is at once an objective and an engine of development. As an engine of development, and within the right policy framework, sanitation can provide an avenue for gainful employment for many. By right policy framework, we mean policies that are in concert with the socio-economic and cultural context within which they are implemented. Sustainability in this case is ensured by the use of technology that is appropriate from technical, management and other perspectives. An example will help to illuminate this point. In Egypt, as discussed in Box 8.1 (Chapter 8), garbage collection in the country's largest city, Cairo, has been the business of the ordinary citizens. Those involved in garbage collection originate in the country's mainly Coptic Christian minority community, and are known as the *zabbaleen*. For more than half a century, the *zabbaleen* have done a lot more than simply collect garbage in Cairo. According to an article in the Chicago Tribune, dated February 24, 2003, the *zabbaleen* have over the years "developed the most refined, entrepreneurial garbage processing system in the world" (Chicago Tribune, 2003, para. 9). The ingenuity of the *zabbaleen* in this regard is attested to by the fact that they recycle as much as 80 per cent of the garbage they collect in Cairo every day. This recycling rate exceeds by a very wide margin the 20 percent recycle rate that European multi-national corporations are barely able to attain (see Chapter 8).

Garbage collection is very lucrative to the *zabbaleen* for at least two reasons. First, it guarantees them an avenue for gainful employment. Second, it serves as a guaranteed source of food for the herds of pigs and other animals they raise for consumption and commercial purposes. In fact, the value that the *zabbaleen* place on garbage reinforces the old adage that "one man's trash is another man's treasure." Cairo residents pay the *zabbaleen* the equivalence of $1.00 a month for their services. The lucrative, hence competitive nature of the informal garbage industry in Cairo was manifested at one point by the fact that Cairo's households were divided into "concessions" by the *zabbaleen*. The concessions were essentially 'waste-mining' claims that have been passed down through individual families (Chicago Tribune, 2003). To further underscore the value of garbage in Cairo, the *zabbaleen* pay as much as $600 a month for garbage generated by up-scale hotels such as those with a five-star rating.

In recent times, and in the name of modernization, the responsibility for collecting Cairo's garbage has been handed to European multi-national corporations. In particular, one Italian and two Spanish companies now charge the sum of $30 million a year to collect Cairo's garbage. This is an example of employing the wrong technology to achieve an otherwise laudable goal. There is no question regarding the importance of keeping a city clean. The question has to do with how to go about attaining this goal. While the hiring of corporations or formal companies to undertake this task may be apropos in Western countries, the Cairo case suggests that it may not be the appropriate technology for dealing with the situation in a non-Western setting. In Cairo, the hiring of European multi-national companies to collect the city's garbage has had major negative socio-economic consequences. The many families that specialized in garbage collection, recycling discarded containers, plastic water bottles, and collecting rotting food as fodder for large herds of pigs, are out of work.

*Social change*

For sanitation improvement strategies and technologies to be sustainable, they must include the voices of the real and potential beneficiaries. Thus, serious efforts must be made to ensure that solutions to sanitation problems come not only from the top, but also from the bottom (grassroots). A significant portion of the hygiene and sanitation problems identified in this book are a function of personal behaviour. Examples include open defecation, littering, and failure to practice hand washing. Resolving problems such as these will invariably require a considerable degree of behaviour modification. More importantly, sanitation has been linked to issues of social empowerment, equity and gender (SSA, 2011).

*Capacity development and knowledge exchange*

Sustainable sanitation entails efforts to institutionalize available sanitation practices, and technologies. The success of such institutionalization depends on the extent to which knowledge and capacity are exchanged on a continuous basis. This requires, among other things, that networks and learning platforms be established at all levels. It also requires some coordination mechanisms for exchanging such information (SSA, 2011). The exchange of knowledge and capacity building can constitute an important basis for informed decision making. It can also provide an important platform for transferring knowledge from one generation to another. More importantly, the exchange of knowledge and capacity in the sanitation domain can permit stakeholders to gain valuable technical knowledge.

*Participatory planning process*

Participation in the context of sustainable sanitation calls for the serious and meaningful involvement of all institutional bodies and stakeholders in the planning process. Such participation must begin with an identification of institutional and individual or group stakeholders. Accuracy in this process depends on the extent to which authorities understand the nature of sanitation. It is above all, an inter-organizational or inter-agency undertaking. Authorities must therefore understand that sanitation overlaps, and is inextricably intertwined with other sectors of a polity's political-economy. For instance, urban planning, public health and education, which are typically under different politico-administrative institutions, are directly in charge of hygiene and sanitation. The failure to recognize this truism partially explains the disappointing results of hygiene and sanitation initiatives in Africa.

Also crucial is the need for authorities to be more serious with efforts to implement extant rules and regulations. The building codes in force throughout Africa already include stipulations for hygiene and sanitation. For instance, ample ventilation is required for all buildings. Furthermore, and more importantly for the present purpose, the provision of improved sanitation facilities is mandatory for all residential, commercial, and public facilities. However, for a multitude of reasons mainly related to institutional ineptitude, these codes are almost never enforced.

*Sanitation as a productive sector*

As suggested above, sanitation can serve as an avenue for gainful economic activity. As the Sustainable Sanitation Alliance states, "the sanitation sector is capable of paying for itself several times over in benefits" (2011: 3). The sustainability of a sanitation system in this case is evaluated based on the extent to which it generates by-products that can be captured and used as resources of their own. The use of water from treated sewerage as manure or fertilizer exemplifies this situation. Sustainable sanitation, therefore, does not view garbage and/or excreta as waste per se. Instead, it is appreciated for the many ways in which it contributes or can contribute to development at the individual, household, and national levels.

*New management systems*

The notion of sustainability in sanitation goes beyond issues that are directly related to the actual technology used in the collection and disposal of waste. It includes the management techniques involved in the process. For instance, there are questions such as those implied above. Should garbage collection, for instance, be undertaken by citizens themselves or by corporate entities? What model is apropos for sanitation activities such as garbage collection? Should hygiene and sanitation activities such as garbage collection be privatized? What management model is preferable—centralized versus decentralized? The sustainability of any strategy can be evaluated through various means. The most commonly used evaluation tool in this case is cost-benefit analysis. Thus, the choice of any given tool depends on a careful consideration of its costs and benefits.

*Innovative financing*

Financial resources are necessary for any sanitation system to function. To be considered sustainable, a sanitation system must operate on a financing structure that is sound and replicable. In fact, everything about sanitation revolves around financial resources. These resources may constitute an input into the sanitation system. They may also assume the form of outputs from the economically gainful activities that can take place within the system. The size of the outputs would depend on the extent to which the system was planned with sustainability in mind. In resource-scarce settings, the absence or scarcity of financial resources typically demand that alternative sanitation methods be sought. Yet, it is clear that no system can function at all without some input of financial resources. Whatever the case, it is important to note that the system cannot be sustainable without some innovative financial management scheme.

## Citizen participation as a sustainable hygiene and sanitation strategy

A perennial barrier to public programme and project success in Africa has to do with resource scarcity. Occasional infusions of capital from the colonial master nations into colonial government coffers veiled the critical nature of this problem during the colonial era. Today, the problem has been exposed thanks to two eventualities. First, Africa's development problematic has grown in complexity. Second, colonialism has since ended. This means amongst other things, the non-existence of colonial master nations. Consequently, orthodox development strategies that depend on resource input from national governments are unlikely to succeed in African countries. Yet, resources are critical for the success of development projects, including those designed to improve hygiene and sanitation conditions. There is therefore an urgent need for researchers, planners and policy makers to craft innovative and sustainable strategies to implement development programmes and projects in the face of resource scarcity. The remainder of this chapter seeks to contribute to efforts intended to address this need. In particular, it advances citizen participation (CP) as a viable and sustainable strategy for implementing hygiene and sanitation projects and programmes in Africa and other resource-scarce settings.

Also known as 'self-help' or 'self-reliant development,' CP, as I recently argued elsewhere, is contextually-relevant, people-centered, and dovetails neatly into African ethos (see Njoh, 2011). More importantly, the strategy contains ingredients that are compatible with post-modern thinking in development. Such thinking frowns on the ambitious schemes and one-size-fits-all prescriptions characteristic of orthodox international development initiatives. However, it is necessary to acknowledge the dearth of knowledge on CP as a development strategy. It is not clear what CP portends in practice. If nothing else, it is clear that, the name notwithstanding, self-help projects often involve more than local citizens alone. Lessons of experience suggest that self-help projects in any given community typically involve entities from outside of that community. Two important factors place these projects under the rubric of self-help initiatives. First, they are conceived and realized by local citizens.

### Box 10.1 A Korean-sponsored public toilet in Bamenda, Cameroon

Bamenda has a population of a little more than 1 million, and is the third largest city in Cameroon, after Douala and Yaounde. Bamenda, the capital of Cameroon's North-West Region, Bamenda has always been reputed as one of the country's cleanest towns. Despite its image as a clean city, Bamenda had no public toilets. This changed in 2009 when the city inaugurated its first public toilet. The need for public toilets had always been on the minds of the town's municipal authorities. However, given their shoe-string budget, the authorities could not address this need. In 2008, these authorities learnt of the availability of funds for sanitation projects in developing countries from the South Korean-based World Toilet Association (WTA) in collaboration with the Government of South Korea. The authorities proceeded to apply for the funds. Their application was one of the 19 out of 90 that were positively reviewed.

Bamenda III Council received a total of US$53,467.12 from the WTA/South Korean government, and added US$13,366.78 of its own for the project. The total amount of US$66,833.90 was applied towards completing the city's first modern public toilet. The toilet comprises two apartments, one designated male and the other, female. Each apartment contains complete toilet facilities including toilet bowls, urinaries, baby cleaning/changing stalls, and provisions for the disabled. The facility, which is located at Mile Two, Nkwen, was inaugurated by the Senior Divisional Officer for Mezam on July 4, 2009.

*Source*: Bamenda III Council website: http://bamenda3council.com/index.php?option=com_content&view=article&id=20&Itemid=40. Accessed, Nov. 17, 2010.

Second, local citizens are responsible for marshalling the resources necessary for their implementation. International development agencies are becoming increasingly prominent as a source of valuable resources for local self-help projects in Africa. International development agencies have grown increasingly distrustful of national governments, and now insist on locating viable local projects to support. The case discussed in Box 10.1 exemplifies this trend in the hygiene and sanitation domain.

Citizen or community participation (CP) has a long history in Africa. In fact, CP is actually rooted in African ethos. In pre-colonial Africa, it was common practice for people in any community to come together to develop communal projects such as the construction of farm-to-market roads, communal markets, and community halls. To be sure, indigenous African tradition does not prescribe collaboration exclusively for the development of communal projects. Rather, collaboration or self-help is a strategy that is employed in any project that cannot be reasonably completed by individuals or households working on their own. Thus, it was common for groups to come together for the purpose of completing projects such residential building construction for their members. This suggests that Traditional African politico-administrative systems practice citizen participation.

The proclivity for collaborative or communal work as an aspect of the African ethos was recognized rather early by colonial authorities. Accordingly, they incorporated the custom as an important element in colonial public works projects. In many colonial settings, the responsibility for implementing hygiene and sanitation policy fell under the auspices of the Public Works Department. Communal work or self-help, therefore constituted an important element in initiatives designed to eliminate shrubbery along roads and streets, unclog gutters, and clean markets and other public places in the colonies.

Contrary to popular belief, citizen participation, especially under the rubric of populism is not an imported ideology in Africa. There are a few instances in which the modern leadership has drawn on the continent's indigenous ethos to implement development projects. Perhaps the best-known of these instances is that of the late President Julius Nyerere in Tanzania. President Nyerere was forceful in promoting the populist notion of 'familyhood' or what is known in Kiswahili as *Ujamaa*. The backbone of *Ujamaa*, Nyerere proclaimed, was the extended family. This, Nyerere believed constituted the basis of what would have been an indigenous brand of African socialism (Khapoya, 1998). Nyerere's philosophy was inspired by the fact that in pre-colonial Africa, communities were organized into well-knit networks of extended families, which embraced a collective ethic wherein critical but scarce resources were communally owned and shared.

Contemporary authorities can tap on this ancient indigenous tradition to address pressing hygiene and sanitation problems on the continent today. A logical starting point in this regard is to divide human settlements, including towns and cities, into small manageable neighbourhoods. These neighbourhoods can then be transformed into well-knit networks by introducing and fostering a sense of communality. Once such a sense is established, shared hygiene and sanitation facilities can then be developed for each network or neighbourhood. Apart from serving as a basis for providing hygiene and sanitation facilities, closely-knit neighbourhoods can also serve as the basis for collecting and managing garbage in human settlements. Sub-dividing human settlements into smaller units as proposed here will invariably reduce the complexity of urban management for hygiene and sanitation purposes. Extant programmes striving to take advantage of African indigenous communal ethos in the sanitation domain have stopped short of actually creating closely-knit neighbourhoods as suggested here. However, the problem of resource scarcity has compelled these authorities to follow in the footsteps of their colonial predecessors. In this regard, national and municipal authorities in African countries are increasingly eliciting 'communalism' as a strategy for executing public works projects. The case of the Limbe Urban Council, Cameroon is illustrative. As discussed in Box 10.2, municipal authorities in Limbe have, under their "Keep Limbe Clean" programme, set one day each month on which all residents must take part in cleaning the city.

## Box 10.2 Indigenous African ethos in modern sanitation in Limbe, Cameroon

The global economic crisis of the 1980s, resulted in a significant dwindling of resources for national and municipal governments in Cameroon. Consequently, many public services could no longer be delivered. One of the earliest casualties in this regard was urban sanitation, particularly the cleaning and upkeep of urban centres throughout the country. The national government was no longer able to subsidize municipal budgets as it had customarily done. On their part, local governments had witnessed a serious weakening of their revenue generating ability. Municipal governments were no longer able to pay cleaning crews. Yet, the need to keep the cities clean had become more urgent than ever. Municipal authorities had to device innovative strategies to deal with this problem. Some of the municipalities turned to indigenous African ethos for possible solutions. One of these municipalities is the Limbe Urban Council. It summoned the African tradition of communalism to 'Keep Limbe Clean.' In 1998, the council enacted a policy, Municipal order No. 3/98/99 of 2 August 1998, that set aside every first Wednesday of the month (from 7:30 am to 12:00 noon) as the 'Environmental Day.' The policy requires every resident of Limbe to actively participate in public clean-up activities. Typically, participants in these clean-up initiatives are responsible for clearing access roads and streets of shrubbery, picking up trash from public parks and other public areas, unclogging drains, and cleaning government offices.

*Source*: Njoh (2003: 187). *Planning in Contemporary Africa: The State, Town Planning and Society in Cameroon*. Aldershot: Ashgate.

Participation of the genre described in Box 10.2 is exactly what provides fodder for the mills of critics. To be sure, CP has been criticized on several levels. A quick look at the Limbe, Cameroon case described in Box 10.2 confirms a criticism often leveled against CP to the effect that it is exploitative. Other critics have characterized CP as 'tokenist, inauthentic, incorporative, and even repressive,' (Smith, 1998: 197). However, criticisms such as these are misleading as they fail to distinguish between the 'use' and 'misuse' of CP as a viable development strategy. When properly used, even the weakest forms of CP have been shown to contribute to the successful implementation of public works projects (Njoh, 2003). As described above, CP was successfully employed by colonial authorities for this purpose. However, what is advocated here is not a return to CP as it was practiced during the colonial era. Then, CP entailed mainly the manual labour input of members of the native population (Nye, 1963). Rather, the brand of CP advocated here requires authorities in the hygiene and sanitation domain to seek to meaningfully interact with, and learn from, ordinary people. In this regard, CP constitutes a strategy for contextualizing hygiene and sanitation initiatives. Such contextualization is necessary to ensure the effectiveness, efficiency and sustainability of hygiene and sanitation endeavours.

The experience of those who have actually employed CP as a strategy for promoting hygiene and sanitation in Africa suggests that the strategy's strengths far outpace its weaknesses. For instance, the participatory Hygiene and Sanitation

Transformation (PHAST), which has been tried in some countries on the continent suggests that the strategy has the following advantages (UNDP/World Bank, 1998). If nothing else, it provides a new philosophy and room for developing clearly defined hygiene and sanitation objectives. In addition, it can help ensure that hygiene and sanitation programmes and projects (Ibid, 5):

- are better focused;
- promote improved behaviours of hygiene and sanitation in terms of usage, maintenance and management facilities;
- raise the need and means for measuring progress and monitoring impact while creating awareness and the need to support these activities;
- provide a new vision;
- allow communities to participate fully, breaking down class and gender barriers; and
- allows for discussion of sensitive issues in an environment where social strata and cultural taboos often make it difficult to do so.

Perhaps more worthy of note here is the following fact. Citizen participation is based on the principle that the development aspirations of any given community can be best achieved by the efforts and industry of members of that community. This view contrasts sharply with orthodox planning doctrine. This doctrine advocates 'top-down' programs imposed by the government or any other entity outside of the local community itself. Communities are more likely to identify with planning policies, decisions and outcomes if they are party to the plan-making process.

The UNICEF experience with Community Led Total Sanitation (CLTS) in Choma District, Zambia lends credence to theoretical arguments for CP in the sanitation domain (Plan Zambia/RESA, 2008). The experience reveals that CP can permit the enhancement of citizens' knowledge of hygiene and sanitation. It can also, through CLTS, facilitate the empowerment of local communities to stop open defecation, build and use latrines with no external input. It is easy to understand the effectiveness of CP in this connection. The key is to actively sought the participation of citizen, and help them to appreciate the dangers and indignities of poor sanitation behaviour. By accomplishing this feat, UNICEF succeeded in triggering enough sense of shame, disgust and feeling of irresponsibility about open defecation in Choma. This significantly reduced the incidence of such actions. In fact, CLTS has as one of its avowed goals, involving entire communities "in collective action to end open defecation" (Ibid: 10). In regions where CLTS has been introduced, local residents proudly point to latrines they have built without external support. In such communities, residents police themselves to ensure that everyone respects basic principles of hygiene and sanitation. This suggests that CP can succeed in promoting a sense of ownership and sustainability of hygiene and sanitation initiatives.

## Conclusion

It is clear that the provisioning of sanitation facilities constitutes, or ought to be, a primordial development objective. The absence of such facilities has several consequences. Prominent in this regard are the serious health problems engendered by poor sanitation, and the indignity those with limited or no access to improved sanitation facilities must suffer. While these assertions are largely incontestable, the fact remains that efforts to achieve gains in the hygiene and sanitation domain have been slow especially in sub-Saharan Africa. This chapter has drawn attention to the importance of sanitation as an issue with implications that go far beyond health. In addition to its direct impact on health, sanitation can also affect economic productivity. Appreciating this line of thought can serve as a logical basis for developing sustainable hygiene and sanitation policies in resource-scarce settings. Sustainability invariably calls for serious efforts to ensure that sanitation systems are economically viable, socio-culturally acceptable, and technically as well as institutionally appropriate. Accordingly, sanitation must be seen as comprising more than technical elements alone. As a development issue, sanitation invokes questions of institutional management, community and individual change as well as economic and environmental sustainability. Success in dealing with the multitude of issues inherent in sanitation requires a deviation from orthodox planning modalities. This chapter advances the meaningful involvement of ordinary citizens, that is, citizen participation (CP), as a potentially viable strategy for resolving these issues. This strategy has several advantages. For one thing, it is contextually-relevant, people-centered, and aligns very well with African indigenous tradition. For another thing, it constitutes a refreshing departure from one-size-fits-all initiatives that are commonplace under orthodox planning.

# References

Abiye, Y. (2009). "Ethiopia: Traffic Accidents, Major Public Health Crisis." Online news item published by allafrica.com. Accessed: Aug. 24, 2010 at: http://allafrica.com/stories/200908031206.html.

Abu-Lughod, J.L. (1965). "Tale of Two Cities: The Origins of Modern Cairo." *Comparative Studies in Society and History*, 7, 429-57.

Acemoglu, D., Johnson, S. and Robinson, J.A. (2001). "The Colonial Origins of Comparative Development: An Empirical Investigation." *American Economic Review*, 91 (5): 1369-1401.

Adedibu, A.A. and Okekunle, A.A. (1989). "Environmental Sanitation on the Lagos Mainland: Problems and Possible Solutions." In Rose, J. (ed.) *Environmental Health*. New York: Gordon and Breach Science Publishers.

African Union (2008). "Statement by H.E. Chairperson of the Commission of the African Union: On the Occasion of the Commemoration of the Africa Day", 25 May 2008.

Agbor, J.A.; Fedderke, J.W. and Viegi, N. (2010). "How does Colonial Origin Matter for Economic Performance in Sub-Saharan Africa." Working Paper No. 176. University of Cape Town.

Alwash, R., and McCarthy, M. (1988). "Accidents in the Home Among Children Under 5: Ethnic Differences and Social Disadvantage." *British Medical Journal*, 296, 1450-1453.

Amin, S. (1989). *Eurocentrism*. New York: Monthly Review Press.

Anderson, C.; Agran, P.; Winn, D. and Tran, C. (1998). "Demographic Risk Factors for Injury Among Hispanic and Non-Hispanic White Children: An Ecologic Analysis." *Injury Prevention*, 4, 33-38.

Annan, K. (Online). "From the Secretary-General: Public Health Challenges Also Affect Development and Security." UN Chronicle Online Edition at http://www.un.org/pubs/chronicle/2006/issue2/0206p04.htm. Accessed: Nov. 26, 2007.

Ashworth, W. (1954). *The Genesis of Modern British Town Planning*. London: Routledge and Kegan Paul.

Ashton, T.S. (1948). *The Industrial Revolution: 1760–1830*. London: Oxford University Press.

Ashton, T.S. (1954). "The Standard of Life of the Workers in England, 1790–1830." In Friedrich A. Hayek, ed., *Capitalism and the Historians.* Chicago: University of Chicago Press.

Austin, G. (2010). "African Economic Development and Colonial Legacies." Revue Internationale de Politique de Developpement. Available online. Accessed: Nov. 18, 2010 at: http://poldev.revues.org/78.

Avvannavar, S.M. and Mani, M. (2007). "Guidelines for the Safe Use of Wastewater, Excreta and Greywater." *Science of the Total Environment*, 382: 391-392.

Awofeso, N. (2003). The Healthy Cities Approach: Reflections on a Framework for Improving Global Health. *Bull World Health Organ* [online]. 81 (3), 222-223. Accessed: Oct. 06, 2007 at: <http://www.scielosp.org/scielo.php?script=sci_arttext&pid=S0042-96862003000300013&lng=en&nrm=iso>. ISSN 0042-9686.

Awuah, E. (2009). "Sustainable Sanitation and Hygiene Delivery in West Africa." Learning and Sharing Workshop Organised by the IRC International Water and Sanitation Centre.

Ayataç, H. (2007). "The Institutional Diffusion of Planning Ideas: The Case of Istanbul, Turkey." *Journal of Planning History*, 6 (2): 114-137.

Ayittey, G. (1988). "Africa Doesn't Need More Foreign Aid: It Needs Less." The Hartford Courant, p. B-12.

Babbie, E. (2004). *The Practice of Social Research* (10th ed.). Belmont, CA: Wadsworth/Thomson Learning.

Bauer, P. (1984). *Reality and Rhetoric: Studies in the Economics of Development.* Cambridge: Harvard University Press.

Bauer, P.T. (1972). *Dissent on Development: Studies and Debates in Development* (1st ed.). Cambridge, MA: Harvard University Press.

Bellows, A.C.; Brown, K. and Smit, J. (Online). "Health Benefits of Urban Agriculture." Accessed: June 19, 2008 at: http://www.foodsecurity.org/UAHealthArticle.pdf.

Bemmo, N. et al. (1998) "Impact sur la santé humaine et l'environnement des systèmes actuels d'évacuation des eaux usées, des excréta et des eaux de vidanges dans les quartiers denses à habitat spontané et des zones périurbaines de Yaoundé." Unpublished Paper, ENSP Yaoundé, Cameroon. Accessed: Oct. 21 at: http://www.pseau.org/epa/epaqppc/rapports/liste_fr.htm#ar4.

Berrisford, S. and Kihato, M. (2006). "The Role of Planning Law in Evictions in sub-Saharan Africa." *South African Review of Sociology*, 37 (1), 20-34.

Betts, R.F. (1971). "The Establishment of the Medina in Dakar, Senegal, 1914." *Africa: Journal of the International African Institute*, 41 (2), 143-152.

Bigon, L. (2005). "Sanitation and Street Layout in Early Colonial Lagos: British and Indigenous Conceptions, 1851-1900." *Planning Perspectives*, 20 (3), 247-269.

Biwater (2010). "Omdurman Water Treatment Plant Turnkey Construction, Sudan." Available online. Accessed: Nov. 10, 2010 at: http://www.biwater.com/casestudies/detail.aspx?id=48.

Blumberg, L. and Gotlieb, R. (1989). *War on Waste.* Washington, DC: Island Press.

BMJ (1914). "Sanitation in German African Colonies." *The British Medical Journal* (BMJ), 1 (2766), 46-47.

Boadi, K. (2004). *Environment and Health in the Accra Metropolitan Area, Ghana.* Academic Dissertation, University of Jyväskylä.

Bonnardel, R. (1992). Saint-Louis du Sénégal: mort ou naissance? Paris: L'Harmattan.

Bosman, W. (1705). *A New and Accurate Description of the Coast of Guinea, Divided into the Gold, the Slave and the Ivory Coasts*. London: J. Knapton.

Bossuroy, T. and Cogneau, D. (2009). "Social Mobility and Colonial Legacy in Five African Countries." Unpublished Working Paper. Paris: Paris School of Economics and Institut de Recherche pour le Développement.

Brown, S.H. (1994). "Public Health in US and West African Cities, 1870 – 1900." *The Historian*, 56, 685-698.

Brown, L.C. (1973). "The Many Faces of Colonial Rule in French North Africa." Revue de l'Occident Musulman et de la Mediterranee, 13 (13-14), 171-191.

Brundtland Report (1987). Our Common Future, Report of the World Commission on Environment and Development, World Commission on Environment and Development, 1987. Published as Annex to General Assembly document A/42/427, Development and International Co-operation: Environment August 2, 1987. Accessed: April 20, 2011 at: http://www.un-documents.net/wced-ocf.htm.

Ceesay, A. (2009). "Gambia: Special Court for Anti-Littering Offenders Soon." *The Daily Observer* (Banjul), 13 November 2009. Accessed: Oct. 15, 2011 at: http://www.allafrica.com/stories/200911130406.html.

Chadwick, E. (1842). *Report on the Sanitary Conditions of the Labouring Population of Great Britain*. (Ed.: M.W. Flinn), Edinburgh: Edinburg University Press.

Chambers, R. (2006). "Poverty Unperceived: Traps, Bias, and Agenda." Working Paper No. 270, Institute of International Development Studies.

Chazan, N., Motimer, R., Ravenhill, J., and Rotchild, D. (1992). *Politics and Society in Contemporary Africa*. Boulder, CO: Lynn Rienner.

*Chicago Tribune, The* (2003). "The Trashmen of Cairo: Letter from Cairo." *The Chicago Tribune*, Feb. 24, 2003. Online, Accessed: April 20, 2011 at: http://www.twentythirdparallel.com/articles/ARABIA_RecyclingCairo.pdf.

Chokor, B.A. (1993). "External European Influences and Indigenous Social Values in Urban Development Planning in the Third World: The Case of Ibadan, Nigeria." *Planning Perspectives*, 8, 283-306.

Christopher, A.J. (1991). "Urban segregation levels in South African under apartheid." *Sociology and Social Research*, 75 (2): 89-94.

Christopher, A.J. (1983). "From Flint to Soweto: Reflections on the Colonial Origins of the Apartheid City." *Area*, 15 (2): 145-149.

CIA (Online). "World Factbook." US Central Intelligence Agency. Accessed: Nov. 21, 2010 at: http://www.cia.org .

Clignet, R. and Forster, P.J. (1964). "French and British Colonial Education." *Comparative Education Review*, 8 (2): 191-198.

Coates, S. (1999). "A Gender and Development Approach to Water, Sanitation and Hygiene Programmes." A WaterAid Briefing Paper. Available online. Accessed: April 20, 2011 at: http://www.wateraid.org/documents/a_gender_development_approach.pdf.

Coburn, J. (2004). "Confronting the Challenges in Reconnecting Urban Planning and Public Health." *American Journal of Public Health*, 94 (4): 541-546.

Cogneau, D. (2009). "The Political Dimension of Inequality During Economic Development." Document de Travail (Working Paper). DIAL: Development Institutions & Analyses de Long Terme.

Cogneau, D. (2003). "Colonisation, School and Development in Africa: An Empirical Analysis." Document de Travail Unite de Recherche CIPRE, DIAL, Développement et insertion internationale. Available online. Accessed: Nov. 18, 2010 at: www.dial.prd.fr.

Collignon, B., Taisne, R., and Sié Kouadio, J.M. (2000). "Water and Sanitation for the Urban Poor in Côte d'Ivoire. Water and Sanitation Programme." Accessed: Oct. 15, 2011 at: http://siteresources.worldbank.org/INTPSIA/Resources/490023-1120845825946/af_ci_urbanpoor.pdf.

Cooke, J.G. (2009). *Public Health in Africa: A Report of the CSIS Global Health Policy Center*. Washington, DC: Center for Strategic and International Studies.

Craster, C.V. (1944) "Slum Clearance." *American Journal of Public Health*, 34 (9): 935-940.

Curtin, P.D. (1985). "African under apartheid", Sociology and Social Research 75 (2) (1991): 89-94; P.D. Curtin, "Medical Knowledge and Urban Planning in Tropical Africa." *American Historical Review*, 90 (3): 594-613.

Davis, D.B. (1999). *The Problem of Slavery in the Age of Revolution, 1770-1823.* Oxford/New York: Oxford University Press.

Davis, M. (2006). *Planet of Slums*. London: Verso.

De Tocqueville, A. (1835). *Democracy in America*. Trans. Henry Reeve (abridged, edited and introduced by A. Hacker). New York: Washington Square Press, 1964.

DIAL (2002). "Editorial" *Dialogue: DIAL Neweletter*, Issue 18 (December).

Dibua, J.I. (2006). *Modernization and the Crisis of Development in Africa: The Nigerian Experience*. Aldershot: Ashgate.

Duignan, P. and Gann, L.H. (1975). *Colonialism in Africa 1870 – 1960*. Cambridge: Cambridge University Press.

ECA (2007). *Relevance of Traditional African Institutions of Governance*. Addis Ababa, Ethiopia: Economic Commission for Africa.

Echenberg, M. and Filipovitch, J. (1986). "African Military Labour and the Building of the Office du Niger Installations, 1925-1950." *Journal of African History*, 27: 533-551.

Engels, F. (1845). *The Condition of the Working Class in England in 1844*. (Ed. & Forward Victor Kiernan). Penguin, 1987 (Orig.: 1845).

Fanon, F. (1967). *Black Skin, White Mask*. New York: Grove Press.

FDOL (Free Dictionary on Line) (Online). http://www.thefreedictionary.com/ideology. Accessed: 26 May 2007.

Fields, B. (1990). "Slavery, Race and Ideology in the United States of America." (pp. 102-103), *New Left Review*, 181: 95-118.

Fields, B. (1982a). "Slavery, Race and Ideology in the United States of America." *New Left Review* 181, 95-118.

Fields, B. (1982b). "Ideology and Race in American History," in Kousser, J. Morgan and James M. McPherson, eds., *Region, Race and Reconstruction: Essays in Honor of C. Vann Woodward*, Oxford, 143-177.

Finlay, A.M. and Paddison, R. (1986). "Planning the Arab City: The Cases of Tunis and Rabat." *Progress in Planning*, 26: 1-82.

Firmin-Sellers, K. and P. Sellers (1999). "Expected Failures and Unexpected Successes of Land Titling in Africa." *World Development*, 27: 1115-1128.

Fox, A.J. and Goldblatt, P. (1982). *Longitudinal Study: Socio-Demographic Mortality Differentials 1971 – 1975.* London: OPCS.

Freiberger, E. (2007). Sustainability Evaluation of Sanitation Projects. Masters Thesis. The University of Natural Resources & Life Sciences (Universitat fur Bldenkultur, BOKU), Vienna, Austria.

Frenkel, S. and Western, J. (1988). "Pretext or Prophylaxis? Racial Segregation and Malarial Mosquitoes in a British Tropical Colony: Sierra Leone." *Annals of the Association of American Geographers*, 78 (2): 211-28.

Frumkin, H. (2005). "Health, Equity, and the Built Environment" (Guest Editorial). *Environmental Perspectives* 113 (5): 290-291.

Gale, T.S. (1980). "Segregation in British West Africa." *Cahiers d'Etudes Africaines*, XX (4): 495-507.

Gandy, M. (2006). "Water, Sanitation and the Modern City: Colonial and Post-Colonial Experiences in Lagos and Mumbai." Occasional Paper of the 2006 Human Development Report. Available online. Accessed: Nov. 19, 2010 at: http://hdr.undp.org/en/reports/global/hdr2006/papers/Gandy%20Matthew.pdf.

Giddens, A. (1985). *The Nation-State and Violence*. Cambridge: Polity/Blackwell Press.

Glassman, J. and Samatar, A.I. (1997). "Development Geography and the Third World State." *Progress in Geography*, 21 (2): 164-198.

Gliddon, G.R. (1854). *Types of Mankind*. Philadelphia: Lippincott, Grambo.

Gobineau, A.C. (1853). *The Inequality of Human Races* (A. Collins, Trans.). (New York: Howard Fertig, 1967. (Original work published, 1853).

Goerg, O. (1998). "From Hill Station (Freetown) to Downtown Conakry (First Ward): Comparing French and British Approaches to Segregation in Colonial Cities at the Beginning of the Twentieth Century." *Canadian Journal of African Studies*, 32 (1): 1-31.

Goerg, O. (1987). "Conakry: Un modèle de ville colonial française? Reglèments fonciers et urbanisme:, 1885- années 1920. *Cahiers d'Etudes Africaines*, 99 (3), (1987): 309-335.

Goldsmith, Arthur A. (1999). "Africa's Overgrown State Reconsidered: Bureaucracy and Economic Growth." *World Politics*, 51 (4): 520-546.

Government of Kenya (Online). Portal of the Government of Kenya. Accessed: Oct. 9, 2011 at: http://www.information.go.ke/.

Green, L. (2009). "Dousing of Street Lighting in Wales – Impacts on Health and Wellbeing." Available online. Accessed: March 17, 2011 at: http://www.apho.org.uk/resource/item.aspx?RID=65662.

Grier, R.M. (1999). "Colonial Legacies and Economic Growth." *Public Choice*, 98: 37-355.

Grier, R. (1997). "The effect of religion on economic development: A cross national study of 63 former colonies." *Kyklos*, 50 (1): 47-62.

Hall, E. (2007). "Divide and Sprawl, Decline and Fall: A Comparative Critique of Euclidean Zoning." *University of Pittsburgh Law Review*, 68: 915-952.

Hancock, T. and Duhl, L. (1988). "Promoting Health in the Urban Context." *Healthy Cities Series*, No. 1, Copenhagen: FADL.

Harrison, D. (1988). *The Sociology of Modernization and Development*. London/ New York: Routledge.

Herbert, M. (1999). "A City in Good Shape: Town Planning and Public Health." *Town Planning Review*, 70 (4), 433-53.

Herbst, J. (2000). *States and Power in Africa: Comparative Lessons in Authority and Control*. Princeton: Princeton University Press.

Home, R. (1997). *Of Planting and Planning: The Making of British Colonial Cities*. London: E & FN Spon.

Hughes, C.C. (1963). "Public Health in non-Literate Societies." In Galdston, I. (ed.), (p. 157), *Man's Image in Medicine and Anthropology*. New York: International University Press.

Hull, R.W. (1976). *African Cities and Towns before the European Conquest*. London and New York: W.W. Norton & Co.

Hutton, G., Haller, L., and Bartram, J. (2007). *Economic and Health Effects of Increasing Coverage of Low-Cost Household Drinking-Water Supply and Sanitation Interventions to Countries Off-Track to Meet MDG Target 10*. Geneva, Switzerland. World Health Organization. Available online at http://www.irc.nl/page/38443 .

ICL (Online). "Slavery and the Origin of Race Ideology." From Richard Fraser, *The Struggle Against Slavery in the United States*, excerpted by the International Communist League (ICL). (Posted online on Sep. 11, 2009). Accessed: Jan. 3, 2010 at: http://www.icl-fi.org/english/wv/942/qotw.html.

Inkeles, A. and Smith, D.H. (1974). *Becoming Modern: Individual Change in Six Developing Countries*. Cambridge, MA: Harvard University Press.

IRP (2006). "From Cairo's trash, a model of recycling: Old door-to-door method boasts 85% reuse rate." International Reporting Project (IPR). Accessed: April 15, 2011 at: http://www.internationalreportingproject.org/stories/detail/866/.

Iwugo, K., D'Arcy, B. and Andoh, R. (2003). "Aspects of Land-Base Pollution of African Megacity of Lagos." Paper Presented at the Diffuse Pollution Conference, Dublin.

Johnston, R.J. (1982). *Geography and the State: An Essay in Political Geography*. New York: St. Martin's Press.

Jordan, W.D. (1968). *White Over Black: American Attitudes Toward the Negro, 1550-1812*. Chapel Hill, NC: University of North Carolina Press.

Kanyeihamba, G.W. (1980). "The Impact of the Received Law on Planning and Development in Anglophone Africa." *International Journal of Urban and Regional Research*, 4, 239-266.

K'Akumu, O.A. and Olima, W.H.A. (2007). "The Dynamics and Implications of Residential Segregation in Nairobi." *Habitat International*, 31: 87-99.

King, A.D. (1990). *Urbanism, Colonialism, and the World Economy: Cultural and Spatial foundations of the World Urban System*. London/New York: Routledge.

Konadu-Agyemang, K. (2001). *The Political Economy of Housing and Urban Development in Africa: Ghana's Experience from Colonial Times to 1998*. Westport, CT: Praeger.

Kyambalesa, M.H. (2004). *Socio-Economic Challenges: The African Context*. Trenton/Asmara: Africa World Press.

Lahlou, M. (Online). "Water Privatization in Morocco: First Lessons Drawn from the Case of Lyonnaise de Eaux in Casablanca." Transnational Institute (TNI). Accessed: Feb. 10, 2011 at: http://www.tni.org/archives/act/18357.

Larbi, H. and Leitmann, J. (1994). "Tunis: City Profile." *Cities*, 11 (5): 292-296.

Lee, A. and Schultz, K.A. (2009). "Comparing British and French Colonial Legacies: A Discontinuity Analysis of Cameroon." Papers Discussed at the Working Group on African Political Economy (WGAPE), Stanford University, 11-12 December. Available online. Accessed: Oct. 26, 2010 at: http://www.sscnet.ucla.edu/polisci/wgape/papers/17_Lee.pdf .

Lewis, R.A. (1952). *Edwin Chadwick and the Public Health Movement 1832 – 1854*. London: Longman.

Lipton, M. (1977). *Why Poor People Stay Poor: Urban Bias in World Development*. Cambridge: Harvard University Press.

Locke, R. (2003). "Nation Busting: The Trouble with Globalism." *The American Conservative*, June 2, 2003, online magazine. Accessed: Oct. 5, 2007 at: http://www.amconmag.com/06_02_03/feature.html#.

Lugalla, J. (1997). "Economic Reforms and Health Conditions of the Urban Poor in Tanzania." *African Studies Quarterly*, 1 (2): 19-37.

Lugalla, J. (1995). *Crisis, Urbanization and Urban Poverty in Tanzania: A Study of Urban Poverty and Survival Politics*. Washington, DC: University Press of America.

Lydec (Online). "Lydec (Suez): Temporary Electrification of Shantytowns – Casablanca, Morocco. Accessed: April 19, 2011 at: http://www.iccwbo.org/uploadedfiles/wbcsd/SuezLydecUNIDOfullcase.pdf.

Maier, D. (1979). "Nineteenth-Century Asante Medical Practices." *Comparative Studies in Society and History*, 21 (1): 63-81.

Mann, M. (1988). *States, War and Capitalism: Studies in Political Sociology*. Oxford: Basil Blackwell.

Mannheim, K. (1985). *Ideology and Utopia, An Introduction to the Sociology of Knowledge*. New York: Harcourt & Brace.

Martin, P.M. (1995). *Leisure and Society in Colonial Brazzaville*. Cambridge, UK: Cambridge University Press.

Massey, D.S. and Denton, N.A. (1993). *American Apartheid: Segregation and the Making of the Underclass*. Cambridge, MA: Harvard University Press.

Mathee, A.; Harpham, T.; Barnes, B.; Swart, A.; Naido, S.; de Wet, T.; and Becker, P. (2009). "Inequity in Poverty: The Emerging Public Health Challenge in Johannesburg." *Development Southern Africa*, 26 (5): 721-732.

Maylam, P. (1995). "Explaining the Apartheid City: 20 Years of South African Urban Historiography." *Journal of Southern African Studies*, 21 (1): 19-38.

McKeown, T. (1979), *The Role of Medicine: Dream, Mirage or Nemesis?*, (2nd ed.), Oxford: Blackwell.

McClelland, D. (1961). *The Achieving Society*. Princeton, NJ: D. Van Nostrand.

Mehta, M. (2002). "Water Supply and Sanitation in PRSP Initiatives: A Desk Review of Emerging Experience in Sub-Saharan Africa (SSA)." Water and Sanitation Program (WSP), The World Bank, Nairobi, Kenya.

Memeza, M. (Online). "By-Law Enforcement in South African Cities." Report Prepared as Part of the City Safety Project (Funded by the Open Society Foundation for South Africa). Accessed: Feb. 9, 2011 at: http://www.csvr.org. za/docs/urbansafety/bylawenforcement.pdf.

Meredith, H. (1812). *An Account of the Gold Coast of Africa*. London: Frank Cass.

Meyerson, M. and Banfield, E. (1955). *Politics, Planning and the Public Interest*. New York: The Free Press.

Miliband, R. (1969). *The State in Capitalist Society: An Analysis of the Western System of Power*. New York: Basic Books.

Moe, C.L. and Rheingans, R.D. (2006). "Global Challenges in Water, Sanitation and Health." *Journal of Water and Health*, 04, Supplement.

Muir, R. (1997). *Political Geography: A New Introduction*. New York: John Wiley & Sons.

Nash, M. (1962). "Race and the Ideology of Race." *Current Anthropology*, 3 (3): 285-288.

Nhapi I, Siebel M.A. and Gijzen H.J. (2006). "A proposal for managing wastewater in Harare, Zimbabwe." *Water and Environment Journal*, 20: 101-108.

Njoh, A.J. (2008). "Colonial Philosophies, Urban Space, and Racial Segregation in British and French Colonial Africa." *Journal of Black Studies*, 38: 579-599.

Njoh, A.J. (2007). *Planning Power: Town Planning and Social Control in Colonial Africa*. London/New York: UCL (University College London) Press.

Njoh, A.J. (2006). *Tradition, Culture and Development in Africa: Historical Lessons for Modern Development Planning*. Aldershot, UK: Ashgate.

Njoh, A.J. (2002). "Development Implications of Colonial Land and Human Settlement Schemes in Cameroon" *Habitat International*, 26: 399-415.

Njoh, A.J. (2000). "The Impact of Colonial Heritage on Development in Africa." *Social Indicators Research*, 52: 161-178.

Njoh, A.J. (1999). *Urban Planning, Housing and Spatial Structures in Sub-Saharan Africa: Nature, Impact and Development Implications of Exogenous Forces*. Aldershot, UK: Ashgate.

Njoh, A.J. (1997). "Colonial Spatial Development Policies, Economic Instability, and Urban Public Transportation in Cameroon." *Cities*, 14 (3): 133-143.

Njoh, A.J. (1995). "Planning and Urban Land Use Controls in Developing Countries: A Critical Analysis of the Kumba (Cameroon) Zoning Ordinance." *Third World Planning Review*, 17 (3): 337-356.

Nuttall, S. (2004). "City Forms and Writing the 'Now' in South Africa." *Journal of African Studies*, 30 (4): 731-748.

Nyakato, V.N. and Pelupessy, W. (Online). "Not by Money Alone: The Health Poverty Trap in Rural Uganda." Unpublished Paper. Accessed: 25 Sept. 2010 at: http://www.capabilityapproach.com/pubs/ViolaNyakato.pdf.

Nye, Jr., J. (1963). "Tanganyika's Self-Help." *Transition*, 11: 35-39.

NYTimes.com (2009). "Belatedly, Egypt spots flaws in wiping out pigs." Accessed: April 15, 2009 at: http://www.nytimes.com/2009/09/20/world/africa/20cairo/html?pagewanted=print.

ODPM (2004). *Housing: The Impact of Overcrowding on Health and Education.* London: Office of the Deputy Prime Minister, Great Britain. Available online. Accessed: 25 Sept. 2010 at: http://www.communities.gov.uk/documents/housing/pdf/138631.pdf.

OECD (2010). *Water Governance Across Levels of Governance.* Paris: Organization for European Co-operation and Development (OECD).

Papayanis, N. (2004). *Planning Paris before Haussmann.* Baltimore, MD: Johns Hopkins University Press.

Pedler, F. (1975). "British Planning and Private Enterprise in Colonial Africa." In Duignan, P. & Gann, L.H. (eds.). *Colonialism in Africa, Vol. IV: The Economics of Colonialism.* Cambridge: Cambridge University Press.

Peterson, J. (1979). "The Impact of Sanitary Reform Upon American Urban Planning." *Journal of Social History*, 13: 84-89.

PZ/RESA (2008). "Report on East and Southern Africa Regional Training Workshop on Community Led Total Sanitation Held at Fringilla Lodge in Zambia (14th – 18th July, 2008), Workshop Co-Organized by Plan Zambia and Regional East and Southern Africa (RESA).

Rakodi, C. (1996). Urban land policy in Zimbabwe. *Environment and Planning A, 28:* 1553-1574.

Rakodi, C. (1995). *Harare, Inheriting a Settler-Colonial City: Change or Continuity?* New York: John Wiley & Sons.

Ritchie, M. (Online). "Globalization vs. Globalism." International Forum on Globalization. Accessed: Oct. 28, 2008 at: http://www-old.itcilo.org/actrav/actravnglish/telearn/global/ilo/globe/kirsh.htm.

Rodney, W. (1982). *How Europe Underdeveloped Africa.* Washington, D.C.: Howard University Press.

Rosen, G. (1993). *A History of Public Health.* Baltimore, MD: The Johns Hopkins University Press.

Rostow, W.W. (1960). *The Stages of Economic Growth: A Non-Communist Manifesto.* Cambridge: Cambridge University Press.

Schilling, J. and Linton, L.S. (2005). "The Public Health Roots of Zoning: In Search of Active Living's Legal Genealogy." *American Journal of Preventive Medicine*, 28: 96-104.

Schler, L. (2003). "Ambiguous Spaces: The Struggle over African Identities and Urban Communities in Colonial Douala, 1914-1945." *The Journal of African History*, 44 (1): 51-72.

Scott, R.; Cotton, A.P.; and Govindan, B. (2003). "Sanitation and the Poor." WELL Resource Centre Network for Water, Sanitation and Environmental Health. Available online. Accessed: April 20, 2011 at: http://www.lboro.ac.uk/well/resources/well-studies/full-reports-pdf/satp.pdf.

Sen, D. (2000). "School Sanitation and Hygiene Education." In WEDC Conference Proceedings. Loughborough: Loughborough University.

Shah, A. (2009). "Sustainable Development Introduction." Available online. Accessed: April 18, 2011 at: http://www.globalissues.org/issue/367/sustainable-development.

Sharabas, A. (2003). Water and wastewater sector reform: the Egyptian experience. In Proceedings of Joint WHO/UNEP First Regional Conference on Water Demand Management, Conservation and PollutionControl, Amman, Jordan, 7-10 October 2001, pp. 157-164.

Sherif, L. (n.d.). "Architecture as a System of Appropriation: Colonization in Egypt." Unpublished online paper, Society of Egyptian Architects 1917 (sea1917.org). Accessed: Nov. 21, 2010 at: http://www.sea1917.org/heritage/UIA-WPAHR-V/Papers-PDF/Dr.%20Lobna%20Sherif.pdf.

Simon, D. (1992). *Cities, Capital and Development: African Cities in the World Economy*. London: Belhaven Press.

Smedley, S. (1993). *Race in North America: Origin and Evolution of a Worldview*. Boulder: Westview Press.

Smedley, A. (1997). "Origin of the Idea of Race." First published in the *Anthropology Newsletter*, (November 1997). Available online. Accessed: Jan. 3, 2010 at: http://www.pbs.org/race/000_About/002_04-background-02-09.htm.

Souissi, A. (2001). "Tunisia: Environment and Sustainable Development Issues." Mediterranean Country Profile. UNEP and Plan Bleu, Centre d'activités regionales. Available online. Accessed: April 27, 2011 at: http://www.planbleu.org/publications/prof_tunisia.pdf.

Soulillou, J. (1989). *Douala: Un Siècle en Images*. Paris: l'Harmattan.

Sowell, T. (1983). *The Economies and Politics of Race*. New York: William Morrow and Co.

SSA (Statistics South Africa) (2007), *Community Survey 2007 – Household Services Data*. http://www.statssa.gov.za Available online at http://www.iwawaterwiki.org/xwiki/org/bin/view/Articles/8%29+CAPE+TOWN+%28South+Africa%29+3.

Stock, R. (1988). "Environmental Sanitation in Nigeria: Colonial and Contemporary." *Review of African Political Economy*, 42: 19-31.

Suresh, B.S. (2003). "Globalization and Urban Environmental Issues and Challenges" in Martin J. Bunch, V. Madha Suresh and T. Vasantha Kumaran, eds., *Proceedings of the Third International Conference on Environment and Health, Chennai, India, (15-17 December, 2003)*. Chennai: Department of Geography, University of Madras and Faculty of Environmental Studies, York University, pp. 557-561.

Taylor, J. (Online). "The Racial Ideology of Empire" American Renaissance. Accessed: June 18, 2008 at: http://www.amren.com/mtnews/archives/2006/03/the_racial_ideo.php (Feb. 2005).

Tearfund (2007). "Sanitation and hygiene in developing countries: identifying and responding to barriers – A case study from Madagascar." Available online. Accessed: April 20, 2011 at: http://tilz.tearfund.org/Research/Water+and+Sanitation.

Todd, T.W. (1921). "Egyptian Medicine: A Critical Study of Recent Evidence." *American Anthropologist, New Series*, 23 (4): 460-470.

TRB (2005). Does the Built Environment Influence Physical Activity?: Examining the Evidence. (TRB Special Report No. 282). Washington, DC: Transportation Research Board.

Turner, J.F.C. (1972). "Housing as a Verb," in Turner, J.F.C. and Fichter, R. (eds.), *Freedom to Build: Dweller Control of the Housing Process*. New York: Macmillan.

Udogu, E.I. (Online). "African Development and the Immigration of its Intelligentsia: An Overview." Accessed: March 18, 2011 at: http://www.africamigration.com/archive_03/FINAL%20EDIT%20UDOGU%20African%20Dev.%20Immig.%20Intelligentsia.pdf.

Ujang, Z. and Henze, M. (2006). *Municipal Wastewater Management in Developing Countries: Principles and Engineering*. London: IWA Publishing.

UN (2009). *Global Report on Human Settlements 2009: Planning Sustainable Cities*. London: Earthscan.

UNCHS (1980). Building Codes and Regulations in Developing Countries. Report of the Proceedings of the 'United Nations Seminar of Experts on Building Codes and Regulations in Developing Countries' held in Talbert and Stockholm, Sweden, 17-24 March 1980. Nairobi, Kenya: United Nations Centre for Human Settlement (UNCHS).

UNCHS (2009). *Planning Sustainable Cities: Global Report on Human Settlement 2009* (United Nations Centre for Human Settlement). London: Earthscan.

UNDP (Online) "Millennium Development Goals." Accessed: March 9, 2010 at: http://www.undp.org/mdg/basics.shtml.

UNEP/IETC (2002). International Source Book on Environmentally Sound Technologies for Wastewater and Stormwater Management. http://www.unep.or.jp/Ietc/Publications/TechPublications/TechPub-15/main_index.asp.

UN-Habitat (2006). "State of the World's Cities." Accessed: Sept. 9, 2010 at: http://www.unhabitat.org/documents/media_centre/sowcr2006/SOWCR%205.pdf.

UN-GRHS (2009). *Global Report on Human Settlement 2009: Revisiting Urban Planning*. New York: NY: United Nations.

UN-Habitat (Online). "Mali: Supporting Water and Sanitation Services." Accessed: Dec. 07, 2010 at: http://www.unhabitat.org/content.asp?cid=3273&catid=214&typeid=13&subMenuId=0.

UN-HABITAT (Online). "Focus Areas: Pro-Poor Governance." Accessed: Dec. 07, 2010 at: http://www.unhabitat.org/content.asp?typeid=19&catid=460&cid=2380.

UNICEF (Online). "West and Central Africa Sanitation Crisis." Photo Essay. Accessed: Sept. 27, 2011 at: http://www.unicef.org/photoessays/48826.html.

UNICEF (2006). UNICEF Water, Sanitation and Hygiene Annual Report 2006. Available online. Accessed: March 19, 2011 at: http://www.unicef.org/wash/files/UNICEF_WASH_2006_annual_report_FINAL_Sept_07.pdf.

US-HUD (2007). *Measuring Overcrowding in Housing*. Washington, D.C.: US Department of Housing and Urban Development, Office of Policy Development and Research. Accessed: 25 Sept. 2010 at: http://www.huduser.org/publications/pdf/Measuring_Overcrowding_in_Hsg.pdf.

Waite, G. (1987). "Public Health in Pre-Colonial East-Central Africa." *Social Science and Medicine*, 24 (3), 197-208.

Wang'ombe, J.K. (1995). "Public Health Crisis of Cities in Developing Countries." *Social Science and Medicine*, 41 (6): 857-862.

Warah, R. (2010). "Slums and Housing in Africa: The Challenge of Slums: Global Report on Human Settlements 2003." Published by Earthscan, Ltd., for and on behalf of the United Nations Human Settlement Programme – UN-Habitat – The Chronicle Library Shelf." Available online. Accessed: Sept. 7, 2010 at: http://findarticles.com/p/articles/mi_m1309/is_4_40/ai_114007082/.

Washington Post (2007). "Traffic Deaths a Global Scourge, Health Agency Says." The Washington Post, Online Edition. Accessed: Aug. 25, 2010 at: http://www.washingtonpost.com/wp-dyn/content/article/2007/04/19/AR2007041902409_pf.html.

Waterwiki.net (Online). "The Wiki for Water Professionals Worldwide." Accessed: Nov. 20, 2010 at: http://waterwiki.net/index.php/Welcome.

WHO (2007). "Economic and Health Effects of Increasing Coverage of Low Cost Household Drinking-Water Supply and Sanitation Interventions to Countries off-Track to Meet MDG Target 10." Background Document to the "Human Development Report 2006." Public Health and the Environment: Water, Sanitation and the Environment. Geneva, Switzerland, World Health Organization (WHO). Online source. Accessed: Nov. 27, 2010 at: https://www.who.int/water_sanitation_health/economic/mdg10_offtrack.pdf.

WHO and World Bank (2004). World Report on Road Traffic Injury Prevention. Geneva: World Health Organization.

Werna, E., Harpham, T., Blue, I., and Goldstein, G. (1999). "From Healthy City Projects to Healthy Cities." *Environment and Urbanization*, 11 (1): 27-39.

WHO/UNEP (Online). Policy Frameworks for Addressing Health and Environmental Challenges. Document No. IMCHE/1/CP4 Original: English. Accessed: Aug. 30, 2010 at: http://www.unep.org/health-env/pdfs/TD-Policy-frameworks.pdf.

WHO/UNICEF (2010). *Progress on Sanitation and Drinking Water Update.* Geneva: World Health Organization (WHO)/United Nations Children's Fund (UNICEF) Joint Monitoring Programme for Water Supply and Sanitation. Also available online at: http://whqlibdoc.who.int/publications/2010/9789241563956_eng_full_text.pdf Accessed: Oct. 2, 2010.

WHO/UNICEF (2010). "A Snapshot of Drinking-Water and Sanitation in the MDG Region Sub-Saharan Africa – 2010 Update: A Regional Perspective Based on New Data from the WHO/UNICEF Joint Monitoring Program for Water Supply and Sanitation." Online. Accessed: April 12, 2011 at: http://www.wssinfo.org/fileadmin/user_upload/resources/1284625893-Africa_snapshot_2010.pdf.

WHO/UNICEF (2010). "Estimates for the Use of Improved Sanitation Facilities." Available online (updated, March 2010). Accessed: April 27, 2011. at: http://www.wssinfo.org/fileadmin/user_upload/resources/TUN_san.pdf.

WHO/UNICEF (2008). "A Snapshot of Sanitation in Africa." A Special Tabulation for AfricSan based on Preliminary Data from the WHO/UNICEF Joint Monitoring Programme for Supply and Sanitation. AfricaSan: Second African Conference on Sanitation and Hygiene Durban, South Africa, 18 – 20 February 2008.

Willis, J. (1995). "'Men on the Spot,' Labor, and the Colonial State in British East Africa: The Mombasa Water Supply, 1911-1917." *The International Journal of African Historical Studies*, 28 (1): 25-48.

Wordpress.com (Online). "Sanitation Updates." Accessed: March 16, 2011 at: http://sanitationupdates.wordpress.com/2008/02/26/west-africa-region-ranks-lowest-on-sanitation/.

World Bank (Online). "Catalogue Sources, World Development Indicators." Available online. Accessed: Nov. 21, 2010 at: http://data.worldbank.org/indicator/SH.STA.ACSN.UR and http://data.worldbank.org/indicator/SH.H2O.SAFE.UR.ZS.

Wright, G. (1991). *The politics of Design in French Colonial Urbanism*. Chicago: University of Chicago Press.

WSUP (2009) "Programme Factfile: Bamako, Mali." (A Report by, Water and Sanitation for the Urban Poor, WSUP) Accessed: March 20, 2011 at: http://www.wsup.com/whatwedo/bamako.htm.

WWF (Online). "The Facts on Water in Africa." Living Waters: Conserving the Source of Life. Available online from World Wildlife Fund. Accessed: Nov. 28, 2010 at: http://assets.panda.org/downloads/waterinafricaeng.pdf.

Young, C. (1994). *The African Colonial State in Comparative Perspective*. New Haven, CT/London: Yale University Press.

# Index

Abdel-Halim, 158
Abidjan, 72, 109–111
Abiye, 85, 213
Abobo, 110–111
Abu-Lughod, 13, 39, 213
Accra, 47, 53, 62, 68, 101, 184
Accidents, 2–3, 85, 90, 113, 161, 213
   in the built environment, 85
   domestic, 90, 213
   traffic, 2–3, 85, 113, 213
Addis Ababa, 128–129, 184, 216
Africa
   built environment in, v, xi, 1–13, 17,
      20–21, 33, 41, 49, 79, 84, 91,
      144–146, 192, 216, 221
   Central, v–viii, 16, 63, 82, 93–103,
      105, 107–111, 113, 115–117, 181,
      222
   colonial, vii, 8–11, 13, 15, 20–27,
      29–30, 40–42, 52, 55, 65–68, 70,
      73, 219–220
   health problems, xi, xii, 1, 3–5, 10, 12,
      14–15, 19, 22–23, 29–30, 34, 38,
      42, 52, 71–72, 80, 85–86, 90, 91,
      116, 146, 195, 211
   North, 53, 60–61, 123, 143, 145, 150,
      214
   Northern Africa, v, vii, viii, 16,
      143–47, 149–153, 155–157, 159,
      161, 163–165, 167
   pre-colonial, 14–15, 20–23, 28, 34, 35,
      207–208, 222
   socio-economic problems, xii, 35, 128
   Southern, v, vii, 16, 55, 60, 63–64, 79,
      119–135, 137–141, 219, 220
   Sub-Saharan, 111, 129, 132, 135,
      143–145, 150, 164, 197, 211, 213,
      214, 219, 223

   town planning in, 1, 10, 12–15,
      39–43, 45, 47, 49–50, 63, 81, 106,
      195–196, 209, 213, 217, 219
   West, v, vii, 25
African
   countries, ix, 10–11, 31–32, 35–36,
      63, 69, 71–73, 78, 81–82, 85–87,
      91, 94–96, 99, 102, 105, 107–108,
      114, 117, 120–121, 125–126, 130,
      136–141, 143–144, 150, 153,
      155–157, 159, 167–168, 173, 180,
      182–183, 185–186, 190–193,
      195–198, 206–208, 210, 214, 217,
      219, 221–223
   culture, 34, 37, 63, 67, 77, 91,
      134–135, 219
      as a barrier to sanitation and
         hygiene initiatives, 134–135
   health conditions, 7, 11–14, 29, 41, 73,
      75, 77, 218
   tradition, 21–23, 32–34, 37, 41, 53,
      61, 63, 67, 75, 86–87, 135, 145,
      175–178, 193, 207–209, 211, 216,
      219
   traditional institutions, 21, 75, 193, 20,
      216
AIDS, 21, 82, 127
Akaki River, 128
Alexandria, 158
Algeria, 60, 143, 145, 149–151, 153, 156,
   182
Allen, 131
Alwash, 90, 213
Ambler Realty v Village of Euclid, 78
   *see also* Euclid
Anderson, 90, 213
Anglophone, 94, 102
Angola, 82, 121–122, 124, 127, 136–137,
   181, 184
Annan, Kofi, 13, 213